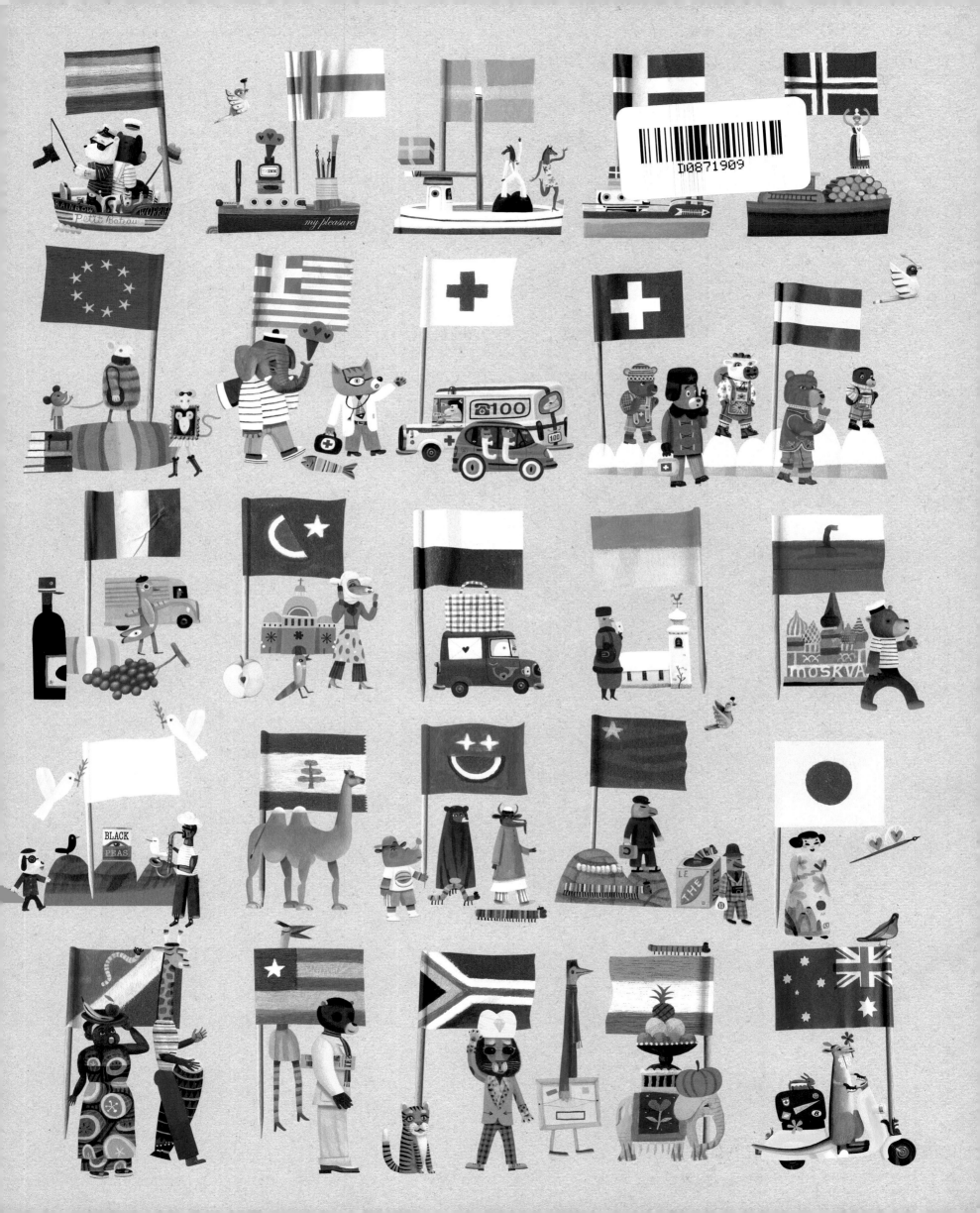

"For my friends,
who cannot always find
the instruction manual."

In this book, Tom Schamp takes you on
a fascinating journey through his world in it,
he combines new material with digital
collages from existing works. This
educational book is just one example of the
many picture books Schamp has created
over the last ten years.

Show & Tell Me The World
by Tom Schamp

Translated from the Dutch by Lauren Napier
and Wolfgang Linneweber

Additional typesetting by Tine Daum
Proofreading by Bettina Klein

Published by Little Gestalten, Berlin 2016
ISBN: 978-3-89955-779-4

Typeface: Nautinger by Moritz Esser
Foundry: www.gestaltenfonts.com

Printed by Printer Trento s.r.l., Trento, Italy
Made in Europe

The Dutch original edition *Het grootste en leukste beeldwoordenboek ter wereld* was published by
Lannoo Publishers. © for the Dutch original: Lannoo Publishers, 2016. © for the English edition:
Little Gestalten, an imprint of Die Gestalten Verlag GmbH & Co. KG, Berlin 2016.

For more information, please visit little.gestalten.com.

Bibliographic information published by the Deutsche Nationalbibliothek:
The Deutsche Nationalbibliothek lists this publication in the Deutsche Nationalbibliografie;
detailed bibliographic data are available online at http://dnb.d-nb.de.

This book was printed on paper certified according to the standards of the FSC®.

SHOW & TELL me the WORLD

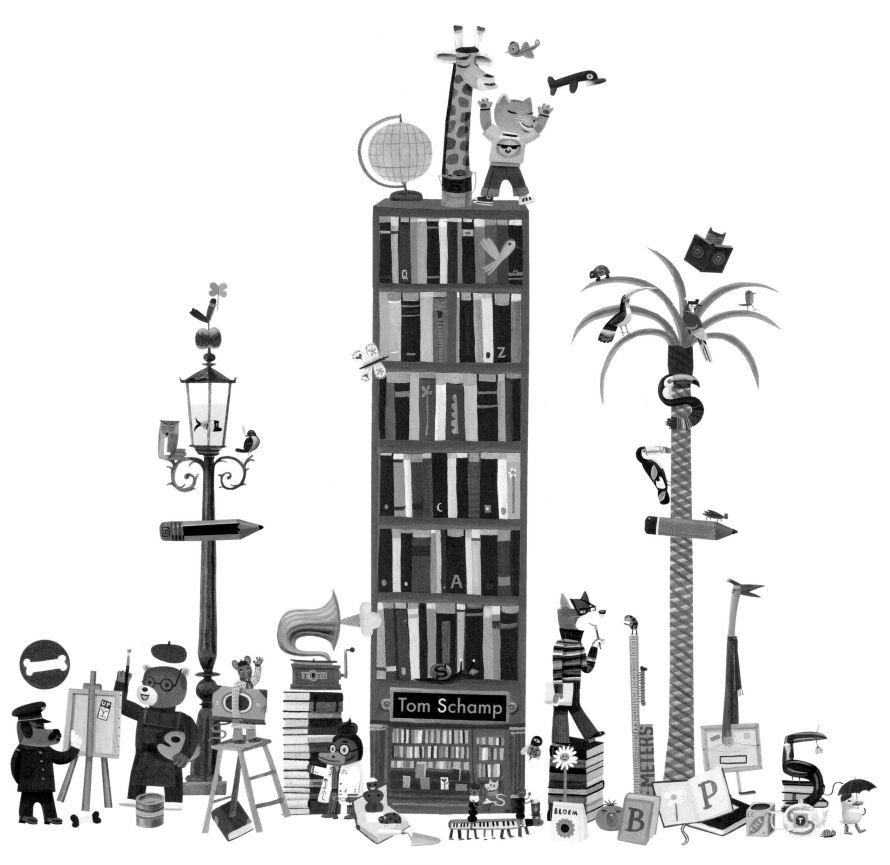

Tom Schamp

LITTLE GESTALTEN

WHO'S WHO?.

Please allow us to introduce ourselves.

This is Papa.

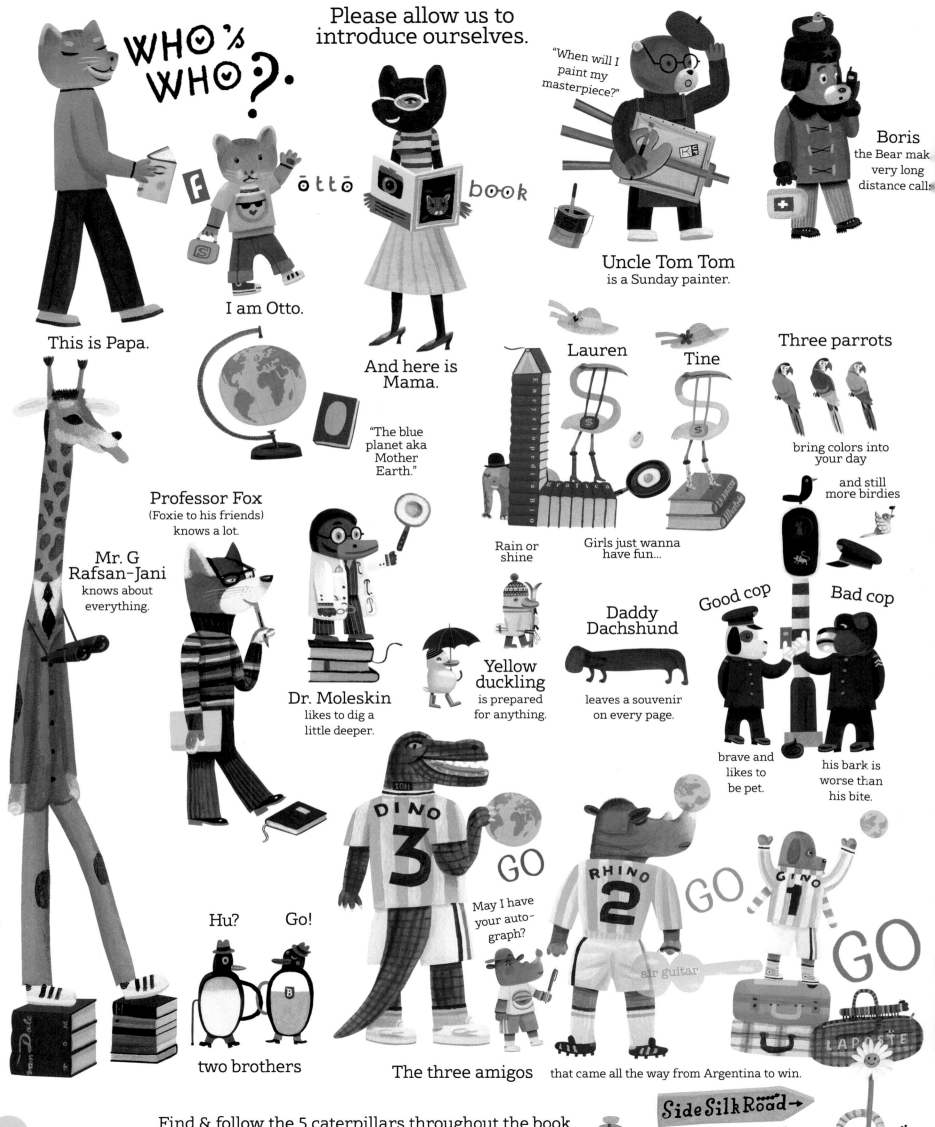

I am Otto.

ōttō

And here is Mama.

book

"The blue planet aka Mother Earth."

"When will I paint my masterpiece?"

Uncle Tom Tom
is a Sunday painter.

Boris
the Bear mak
very long
distance call:

Lauren   Tine

Three parrots

bring colors into
your day

and still
more birdies

Mr. G
Rafsan-Jani
knows about
everything.

Professor Fox
(Foxie to his friends)
knows a lot.

Rain or
shine

Girls just wanna
have fun...

Dr. Moleskin
likes to dig a
little deeper.

Yellow
duckling
is prepared
for anything.

Daddy
Dachshund

leaves a souvenir
on every page.

Good cop

Bad cop

brave and
likes to
be pet.

his bark is
worse than
his bite.

Hu?   Go!

DINO
3

GO

May I have
your auto-
graph?

RHINO
2

GO

air guitar

GINO
1

GO

two brothers

The three amigos   that came all the way from Argentina to win.

Side Silk Road

Find & follow the 5 caterpillars throughout the book.

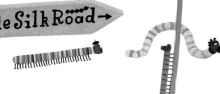

silly silk road

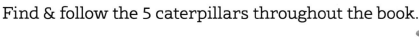

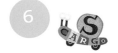

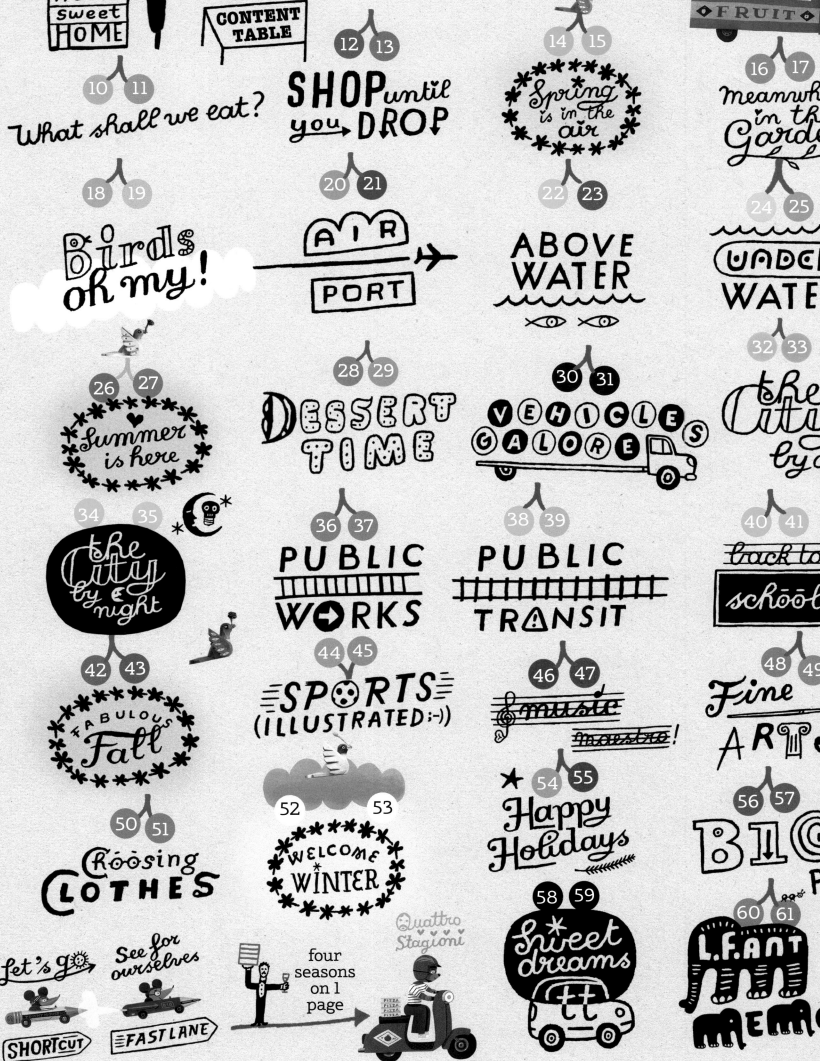

8 9
HOME sweet HOME

10 11
What shall we eat?

CONTENT TABLE

Show & tell me THE WORLD

12 13
SHOP until you DROP

14 15
Spring is in the air

ONE YEAR IN THE LIFE
FRUIT

16 17
meanwhile in the Garden

18 19
Birds oh my!

20 21
AIR PORT

22 23
ABOVE WATER

24 25
UNDER WATER
I'd like to be

26 27
Summer is here

28 29
DESSERT TIME

30 31
VEHICLES GALORE

32 33
the City by day

34 35
the City by night

36 37
PUBLIC WORKS

38 39
PUBLIC TRANSIT

40 41
back to school

42 43
FABULOUS Fall

44 45
SPORTS (ILLUSTRATED ;-))

46 47
music maestro!

48 49
Fine ARTS

50 51
Choosing Clothes

52 53
WELCOME WINTER

Quattro Stagioni

four seasons on 1 page

54 55
Happy Holidays

56 57
BIG PARTY
NEW YEAR

58 59
Sweet dreams

60 61
L.F.ANT MEMORY

Let's go
SHORTCUT

See for ourselves
FAST LANE

S CARGO 7

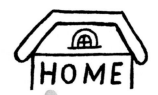
HOME

means something **different** to everyone.

It may be naught to peek in people's houses, but here we will do it anyway.

"This house is not a hotel."

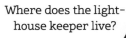

Where does the light-house keeper live?

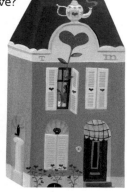

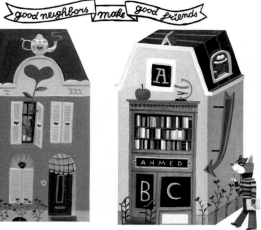

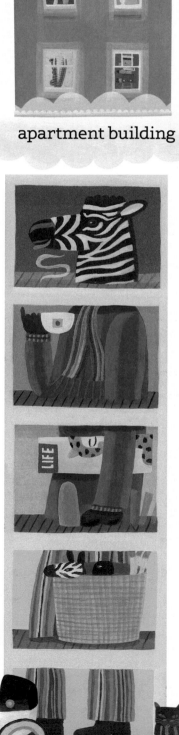

HOTEL

BREAKFAST

birdhouse

hut

pizza house

dog house

dog fence

All over the world people and animals build houses.

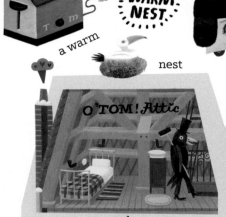

EAST →
← WEST
HOME →
← NEST

a warm

WARM NEST

nest

pagoda

Some people live completely **alone** in a house.

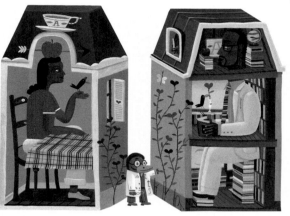

Ms. Neighbor   **Mr. Neighbor**

apartment building

Others live with **many** people in one big building.

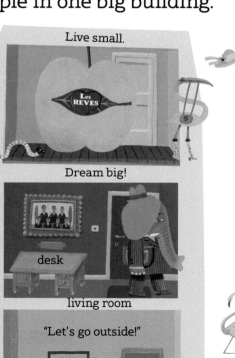

O'TOM! Attic

Hooray, a party!!
C'est party

Live small.
LES REVES

study   **bedroom**   Dream big!

C'est parti

desk

living room

"Home is where the heart is."

What's for dinner?

"Let's go outside!"

another party   **kitchen**

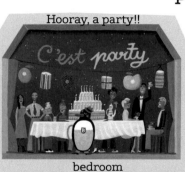
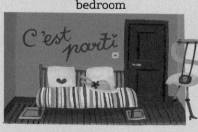
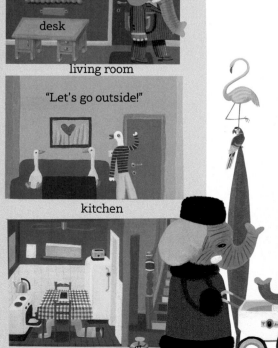

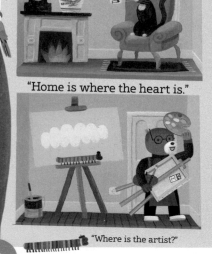

"Where is the artist?"

BABY PARTY

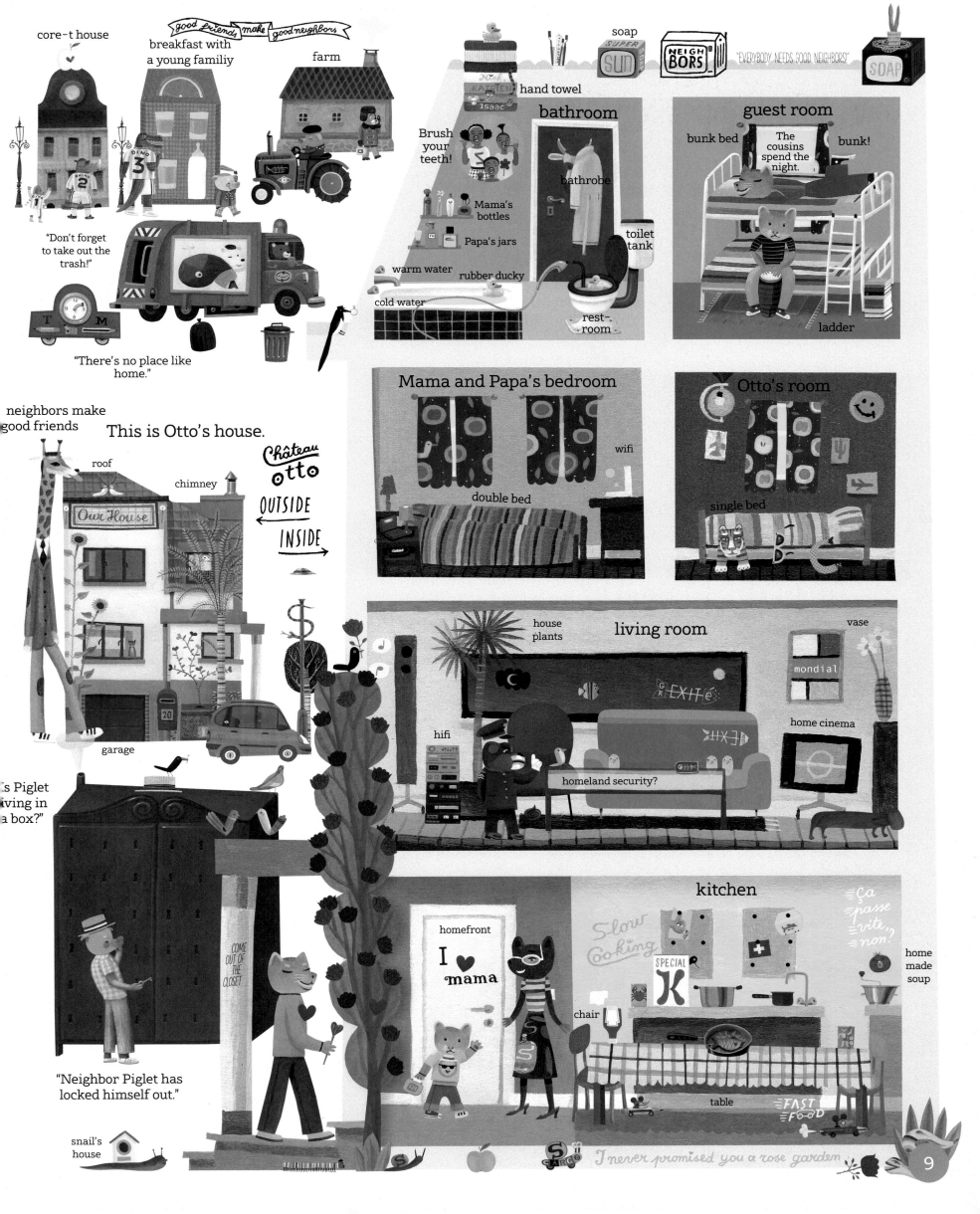

core-t house

good friends make good neighbors

breakfast with a young familiy

farm

"Don't forget to take out the trash!"

"There's no place like home."

neighbors make good friends

This is Otto's house.

roof

chimney

Our House

Château otto

OUTSIDE
INSIDE

garage

"Is Piglet living in a box?"

"Neighbor Piglet has locked himself out."

snail's house

COME OUT OF THE CLOSET

soap

SUPER SUN

NEIGH BORS

"EVERYBODY NEEDS GOOD NEIGHBORS!"

SOAP

hand towel

bathroom

Brush your teeth!

Mama's bottles

Papa's jars

warm water

cold water

rubber ducky

bathrobe

toilet tank

rest-room

guest room

bunk bed

The cousins spend the night.

bunk!

ladder

Mama and Papa's bedroom

wifi

double bed

Otto's room

single bed

living room

house plants

vase

mondial

home cinema

hifi

homeland security?

kitchen

homefront

I ♥ mama

Slow Cooking

SPECIAL K

ça passe vite, non?

home made soup

chair

table

FAST FOOD

I never promised you a rose garden

9

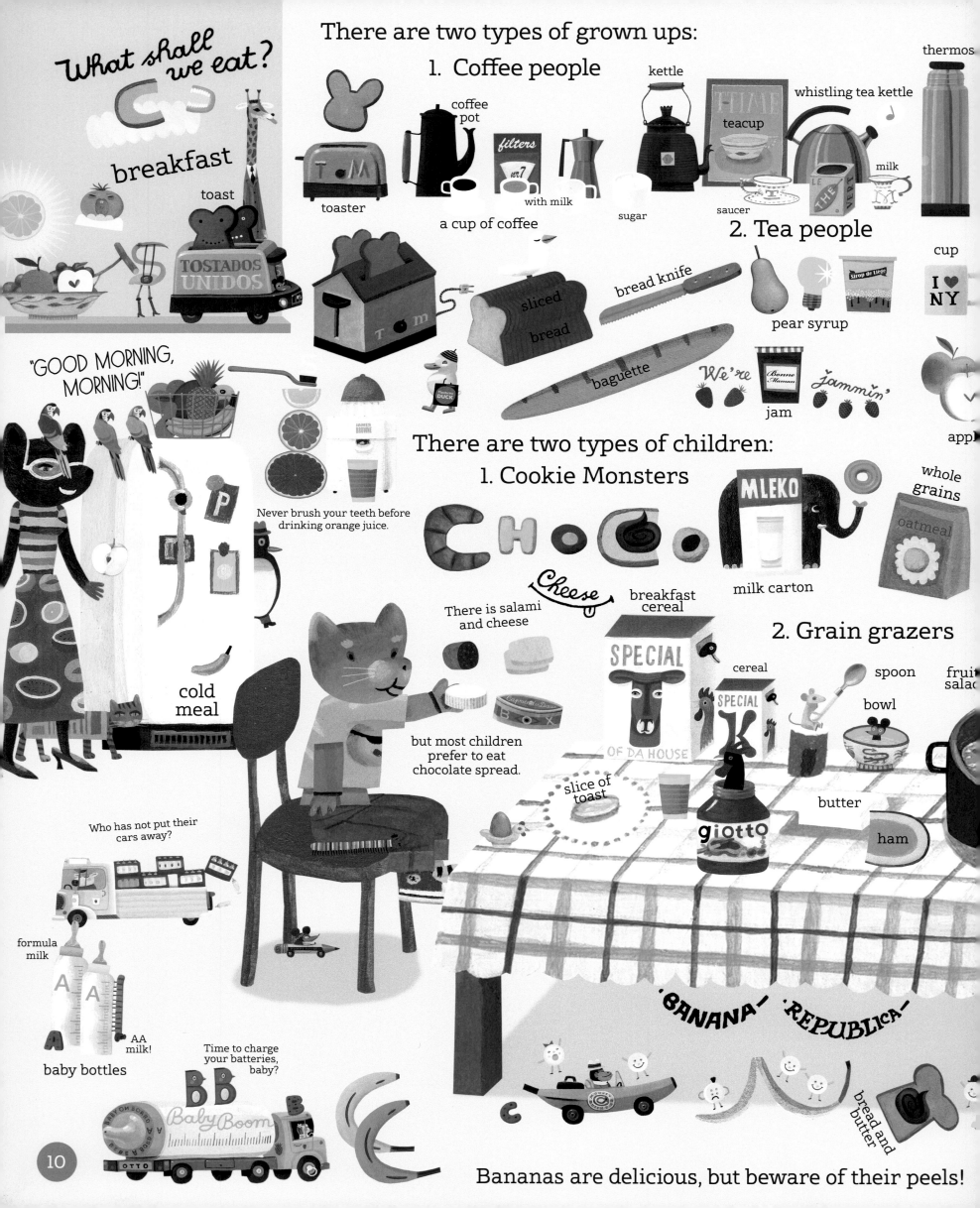

What shall we eat?

breakfast

toast

TOSTADOS UNIDOS

There are two types of grown ups:

1. Coffee people

toaster

coffee pot

filters nr7

with milk

a cup of coffee

sugar

kettle

teacup

HIME

whistling tea kettle

thermos

saucer

milk

THE VERT

cup

I ♥ NY

2. Tea people

"GOOD MORNING, MORNING!"

Never brush your teeth before drinking orange juice.

JAMES BROWNE

bread knife

sliced bread

baguette

pear syrup

Sirop de Liège

We're Jammin'

Bonne Maman

jam

apple

cold meal

There is salami and cheese

Cheese

but most children prefer to eat chocolate spread.

There are two types of children:

1. Cookie Monsters

CHOCO

MLEKO

milk carton

breakfast cereal

whole grains

oatmeal

2. Grain grazers

SPECIAL OF DA HOUSE

SPECIAL

cereal

spoon

bowl

fruit salad

slice of toast

giotto

butter

ham

Who has not put their cars away?

formula milk

AA milk!

baby bottles

Time to charge your batteries, baby?

BB BB Baby Boom

OTTO

·BANANA· ·REPUBLICA·

bread and butter

Bananas are delicious, but beware of their peels!

10

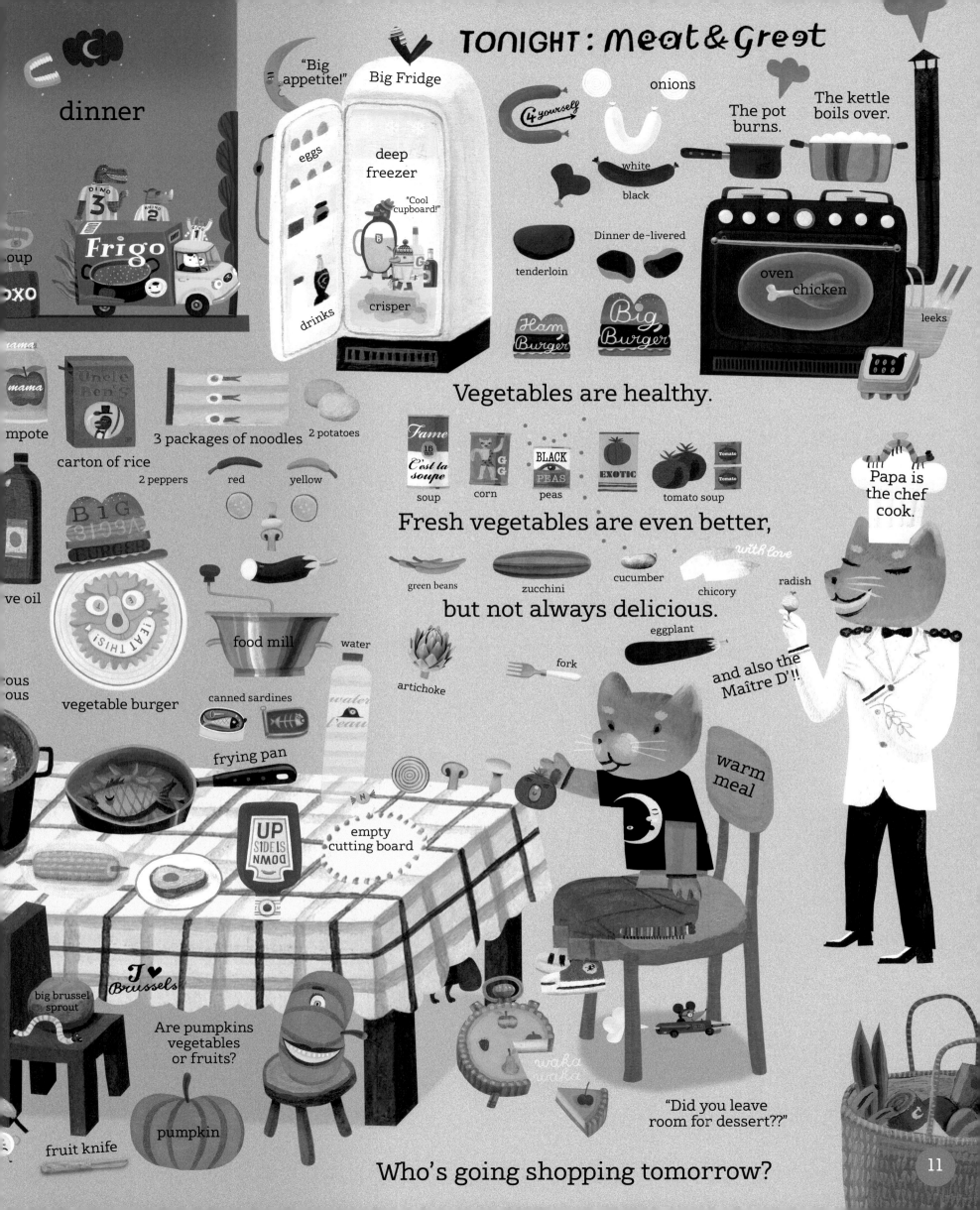

dinner

TONIGHT : meat & greet

"Big appetite!" Big Fridge

onions

4 yourself

The pot burns.

The kettle boils over.

eggs

deep freezer

"Cool cupboard!"

white

black

tenderloin

Dinner de-livered

oven chicken

leeks

drinks

crisper

Ham Burger

Big Burger

Frigo

OXO

oup

Vegetables are healthy.

Uncle Ben's

3 packages of noodles

2 potatoes

Fame 15 min C'est la soupe

corn

BLACK PEAS

EXOTIC

Tomato

Tomato

Papa is the chef cook.

mama

mpote

carton of rice

2 peppers

red

yellow

soup

peas

tomato soup

ve oil

Fresh vegetables are even better,

with love

green beans

zucchini

cucumber

chicory

radish

eggplant

but not always delicious.

food mill

water

fork

and also the Maître D'!!

ous ous

vegetable burger

canned sardines

water l'eau

artichoke

frying pan

warm meal

UP SIDE IS DOWN

empty cutting board

I ♥ Brussels

big brussel sprout

Are pumpkins vegetables or fruits?

"Did you leave room for dessert??"

fruit knife

pumpkin

Who's going shopping tomorrow?

SHOP until you DROP

POP UP · SHOP

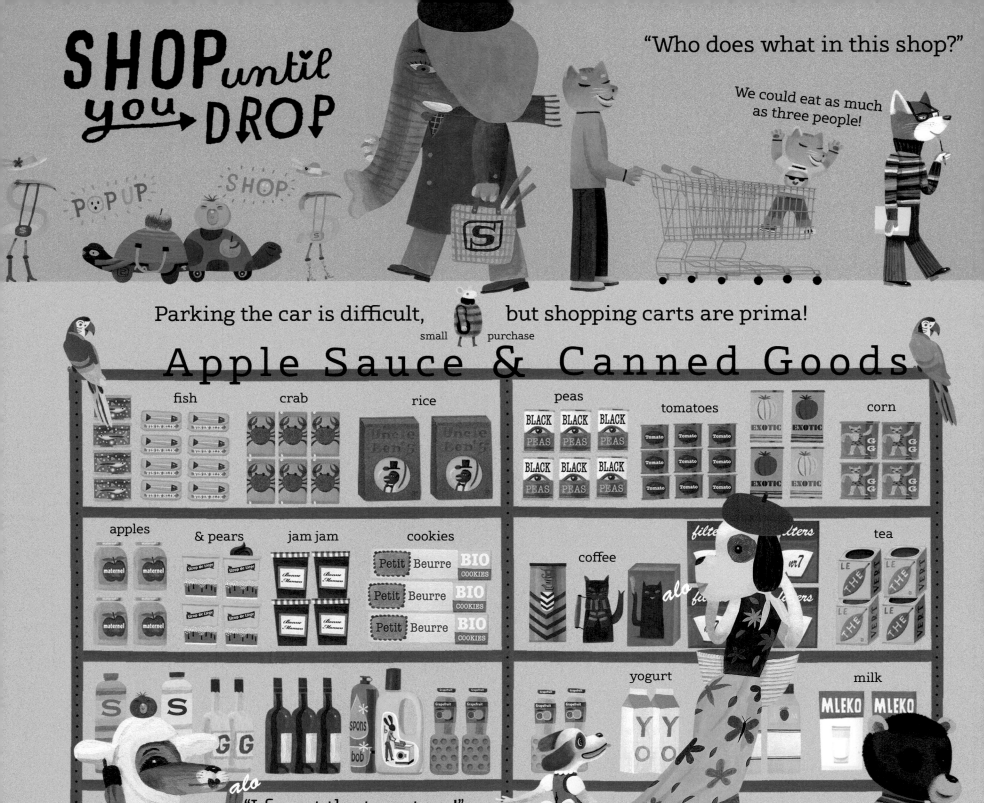

Parking the car is difficult, but shopping carts are prima!

small purchase

Apple Sauce & Canned Goods

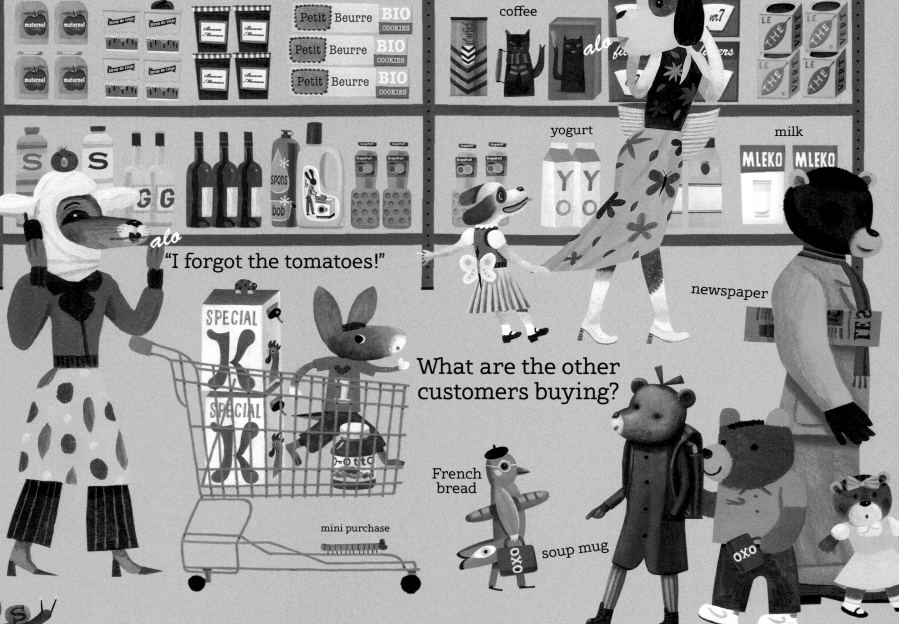

fish · crab · rice

peas · tomatoes · corn

BLACK PEAS · Tomato · EXOTIC · G G

apples · & pears · jam jam · cookies

coffee · filters · tea

maternel · Sirop de Liège · Bonne Maman · Petit Beurre BIO COOKIES

LE THÉ VERT

S O S · G G · SPONS · bob · Grapefruit

yogurt · milk

Y Y O O · MLEKO MLEKO

alo "I forgot the tomatoes!"

newspaper

SPECIAL K · SPECIAL K · otto

What are the other customers buying?

French bread

oxo

soup mug

mini purchase

oxo

12

Oh no! There's already a long line at the cash register.

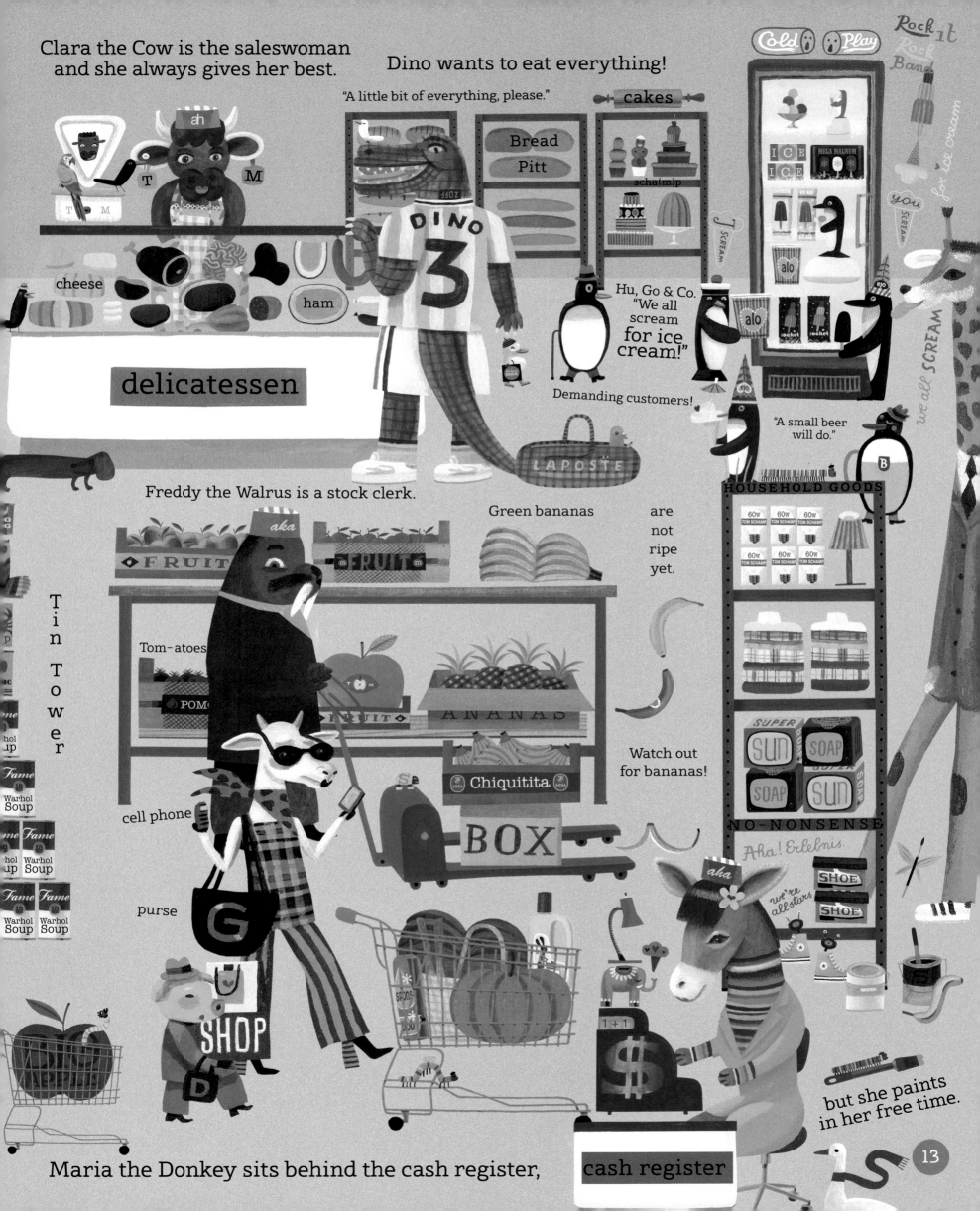

Clara the Cow is the saleswoman and she always gives her best.

Dino wants to eat everything!

"A little bit of everything, please."

cakes

Bread Pitt

cheese

ham

delicatessen

Hu, Go & Co. "We all scream for ice cream!"

Demanding customers!

"A small beer will do."

Freddy the Walrus is a stock clerk.

Green bananas are not ripe yet.

HOUSEHOLD GOODS

Tin Tower

Tom-atoes

Watch out for bananas!

cell phone

Chiquitita

BOX

NO-NONSENSE

purse

SHOP

but she paints in her free time.

Maria the Donkey sits behind the cash register,

cash register

13

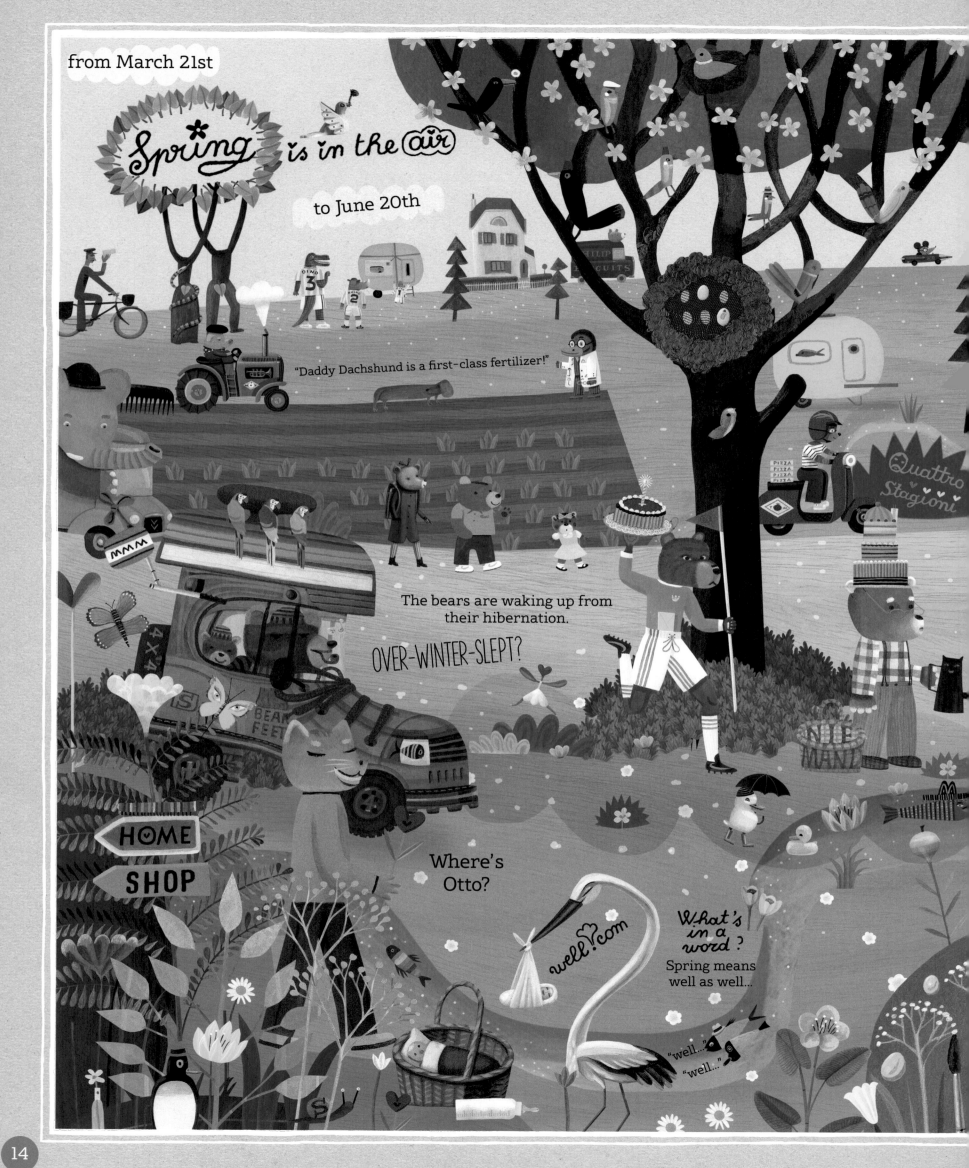

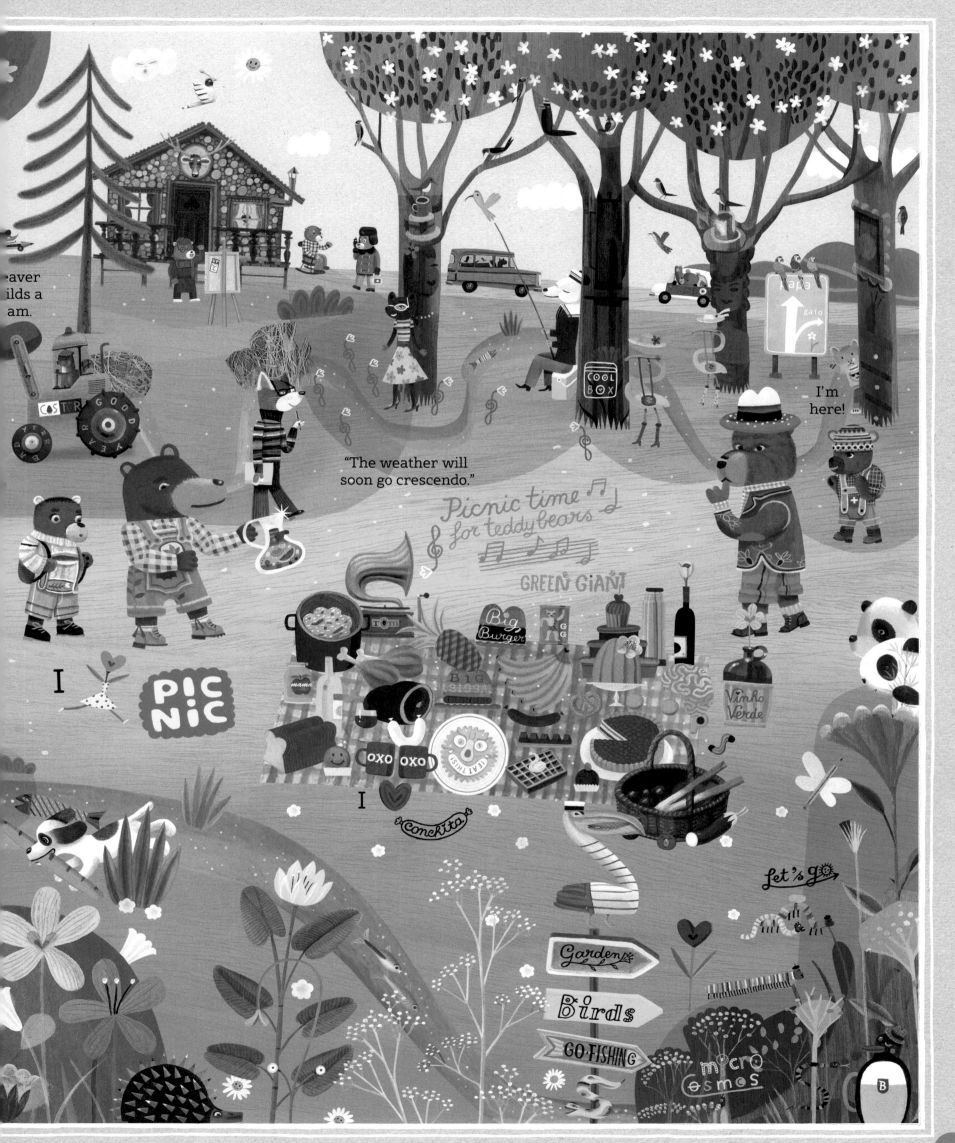

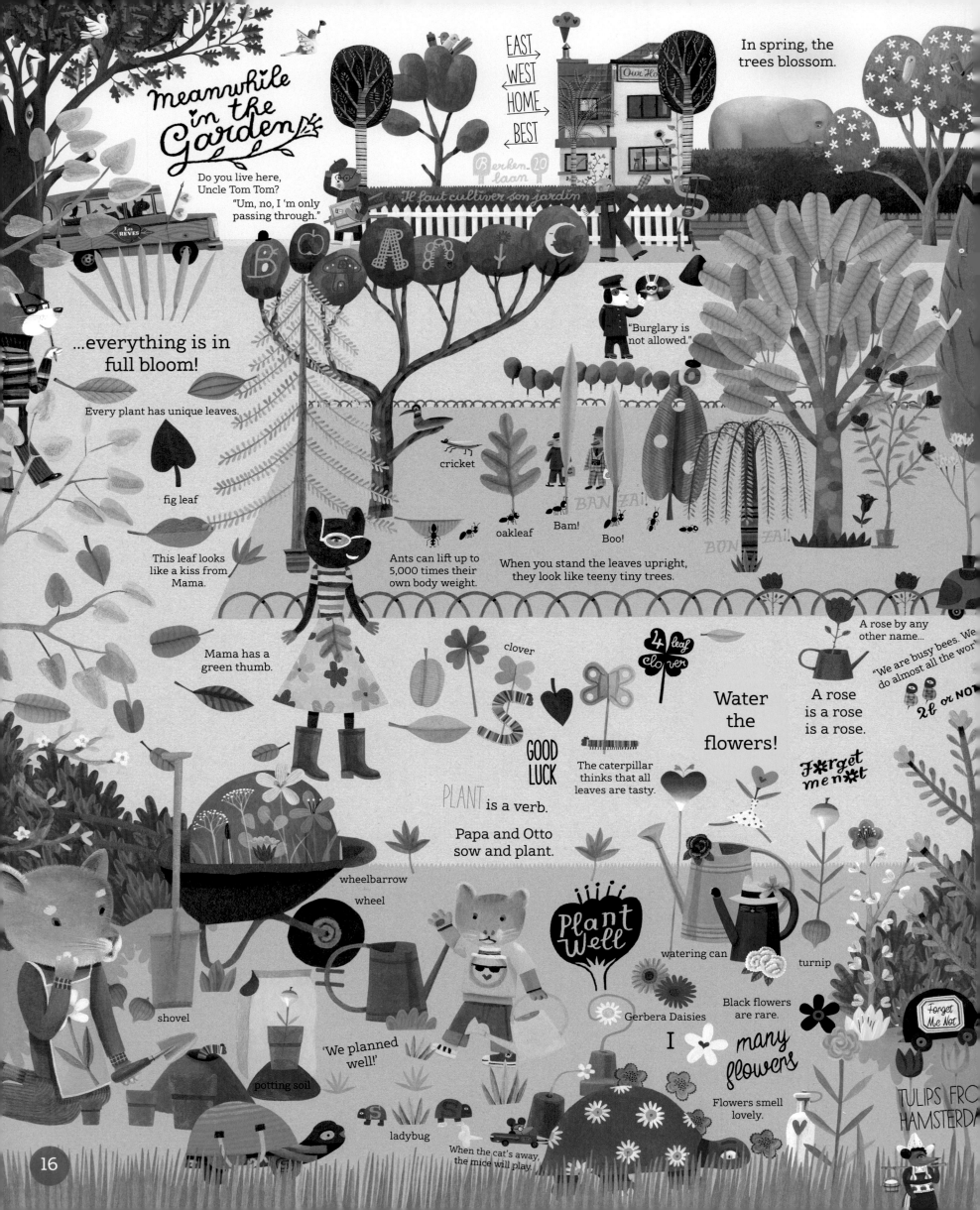

meanwhile in the Garden

Do you live here, Uncle Tom Tom?
"Um, no, I'm only passing through."

EAST
WEST
HOME
BEST

In spring, the trees blossom.

"Burglary is not allowed."

...everything is in full bloom!

Every plant has unique leaves.

fig leaf

This leaf looks like a kiss from Mama.

cricket

oakleaf

Bam!

Boo!

Ants can lift up to 5,000 times their own body weight.

When you stand the leaves upright, they look like teeny tiny trees.

Mama has a green thumb.

clover

4 leaf clover

A rose by any other name...

"We are busy bees. We do almost all the wor"

2b or NOT

Water the flowers!

A rose is a rose is a rose.

Forget me not

GOOD LUCK

The caterpillar thinks that all leaves are tasty.

PLANT is a verb.

Papa and Otto sow and plant.

wheelbarrow

wheel

Plant Well

watering can

turnip

shovel

'We planned well!'

Gerbera Daisies

Black flowers are rare.

I ❤ many flowers

potting soil

Forget Me Not

ladybug

When the cat's away, the mice will play.

Flowers smell lovely.

TULIPS FRO HAMSTERD

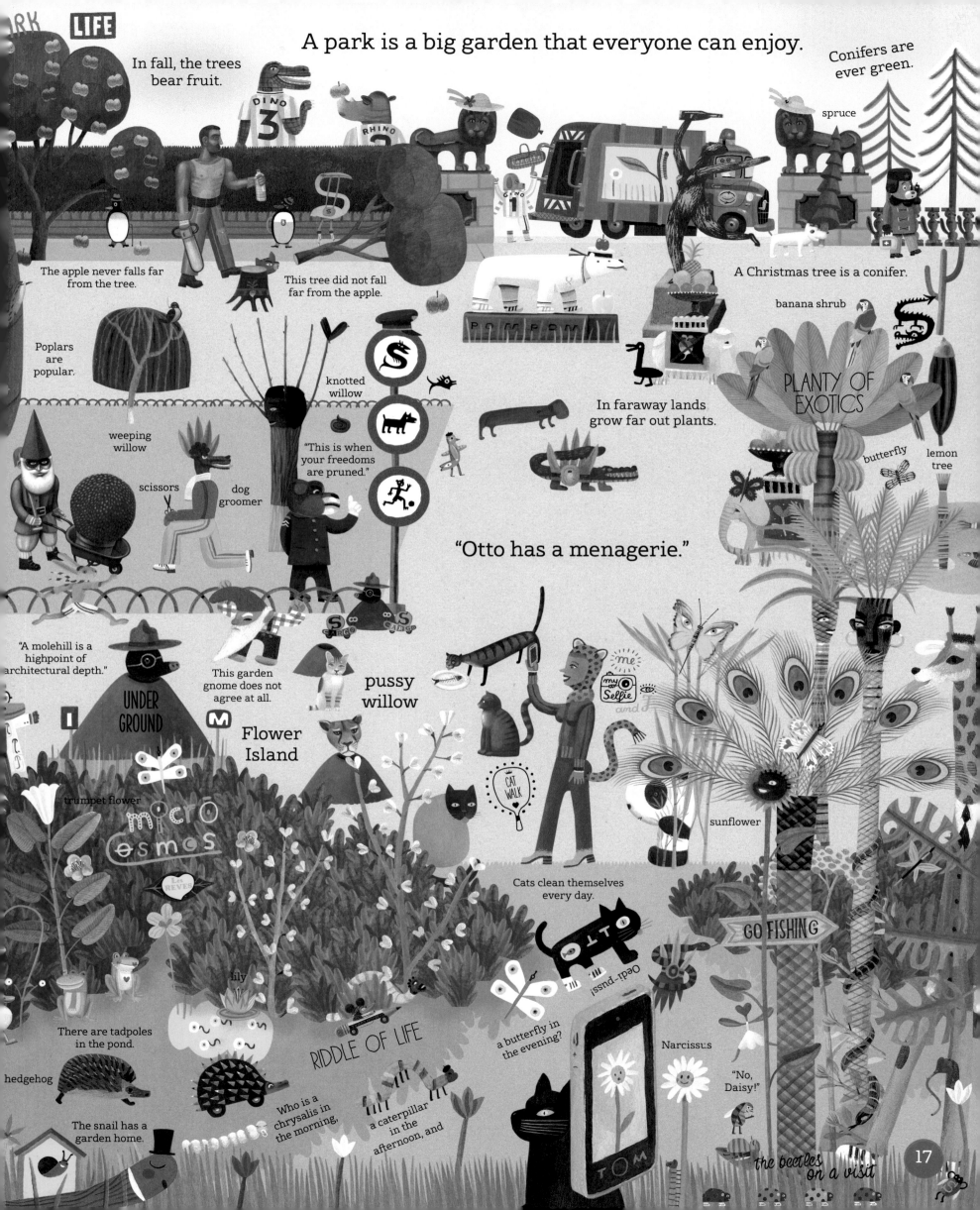

A park is a big garden that everyone can enjoy.

In fall, the trees bear fruit.

Conifers are ever green.

spruce

The apple never falls far from the tree.

This tree did not fall far from the apple.

A Christmas tree is a conifer.

banana shrub

Poplars are popular.

PLANTY OF EXOTICS

knotted willow

weeping willow

"This is when your freedoms are pruned."

butterfly

lemon tree

scissors

dog groomer

In faraway lands grow far out plants.

"Otto has a menagerie."

"A molehill is a highpoint of architectural depth."

UNDER GROUND

This garden gnome does not agree at all.

pussy willow

Flower Island

micro cosmos

trumpet flower

CAT WALK

me Selfie and

sunflower

Cats clean themselves every day.

Les REVES

GO FISHING

lily

RIDDLE OF LIFE

There are tadpoles in the pond.

a butterfly in the evening?

Narcissus

"No, Daisy!"

hedgehog

Who is a chrysalis in the morning,

a caterpillar in the afternoon, and

The snail has a garden home.

the beetles on a visit

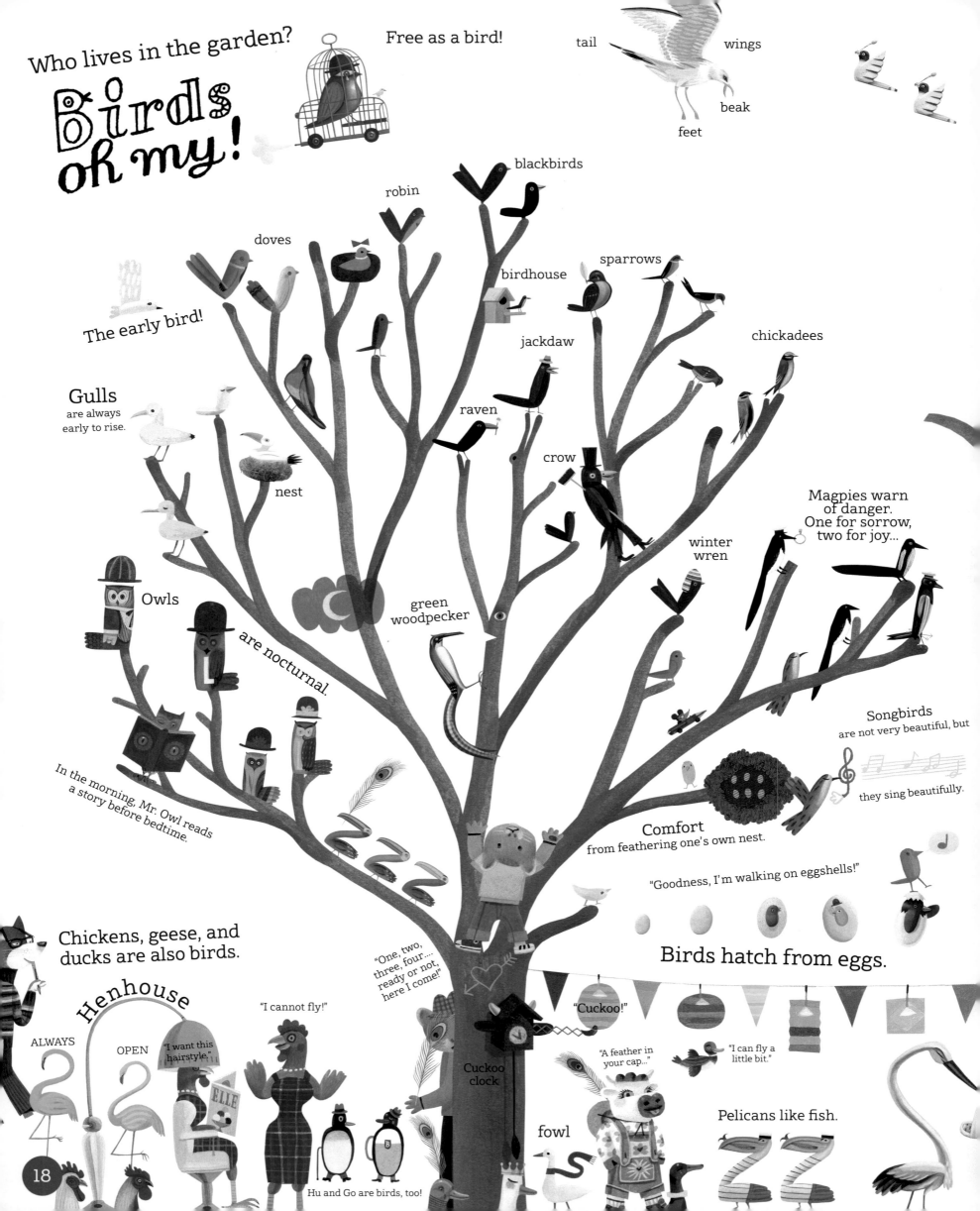

Who lives in the garden?

Birds oh my!

Free as a bird!

tail

wings

beak

feet

blackbirds

robin

doves

birdhouse

sparrows

The early bird!

jackdaw

chickadees

Gulls
are always
early to rise.

raven

crow

Magpies warn
of danger.
One for sorrow,
two for joy...

nest

winter
wren

Owls

green
woodpecker

Songbirds
are not very beautiful, but

are nocturnal.

they sing beautifully.

In the morning, Mr. Owl reads
a story before bedtime.

Comfort
from feathering one's own nest.

"Goodness, I'm walking on eggshells!"

Chickens, geese, and
ducks are also birds.

"One, two, four...
three, four...
ready or not,
here I come!"

Birds hatch from eggs.

Henhouse

"I cannot fly!"

"Cuckoo!"

ALWAYS

OPEN

"I want this
hairstyle."

ELLE

Cuckoo
clock

"A feather in
your cap..."

"I can fly a
little bit."

18

fowl

Pelicans like fish.

Hu and Go are birds, too!

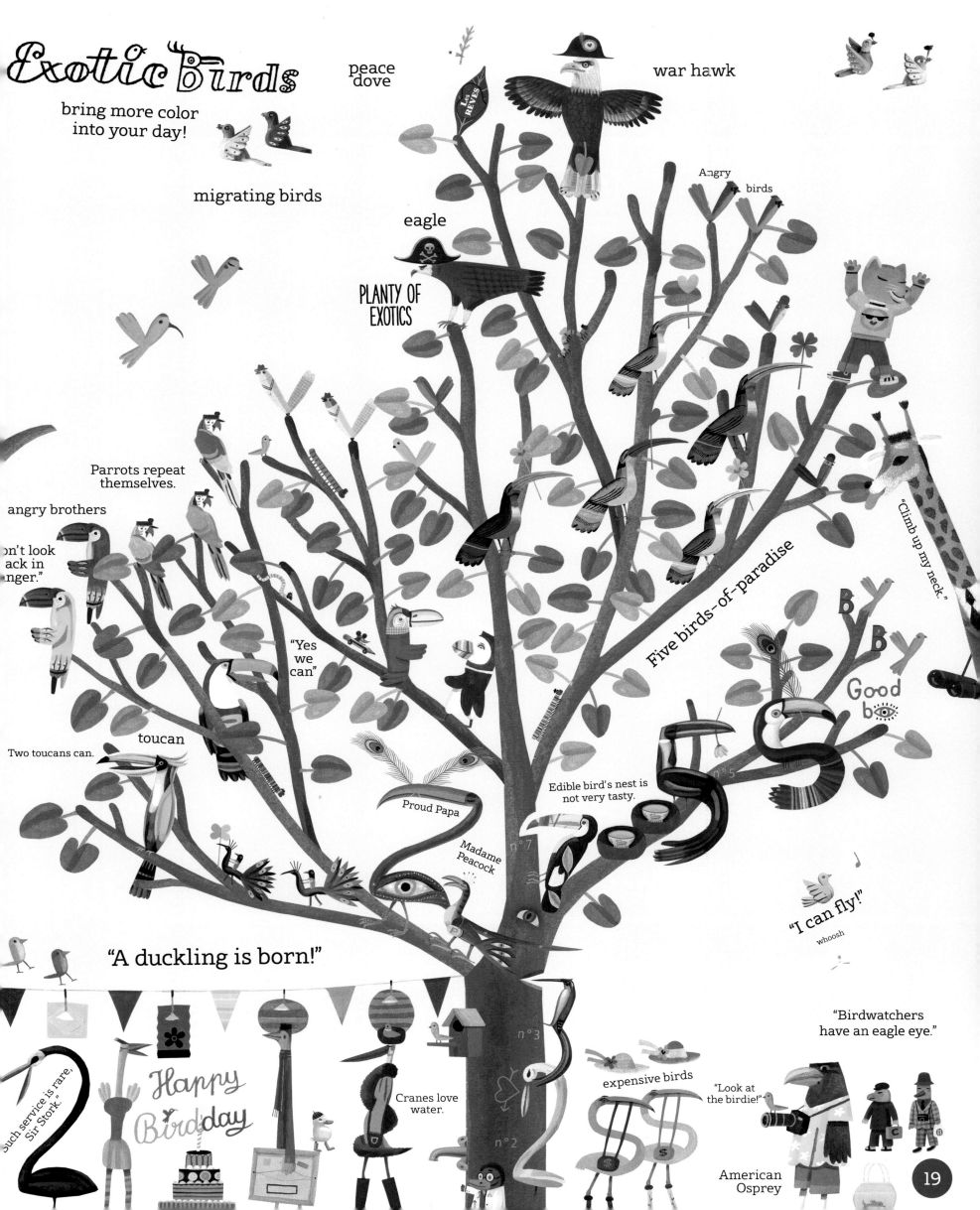

Exotic Birds

bring more color into your day!

migrating birds

peace dove

war hawk

eagle

Angry birds

PLANTY OF EXOTICS

Parrots repeat themselves.

angry brothers

"Don't look back in anger."

"Yes we can"

Five birds-of-paradise

"Climb up my neck."

B B Y

Good bye

toucan

Two toucans can.

Proud Papa

Madame Peacock

Edible bird's nest is not very tasty.

"I can fly!"

whoosh

"A duckling is born!"

"Birdwatchers have an eagle eye."

"Such service is rare, Sir Stork."

Happy Birdday

Cranes love water.

expensive birds

"Look at the birdie!"

American Osprey

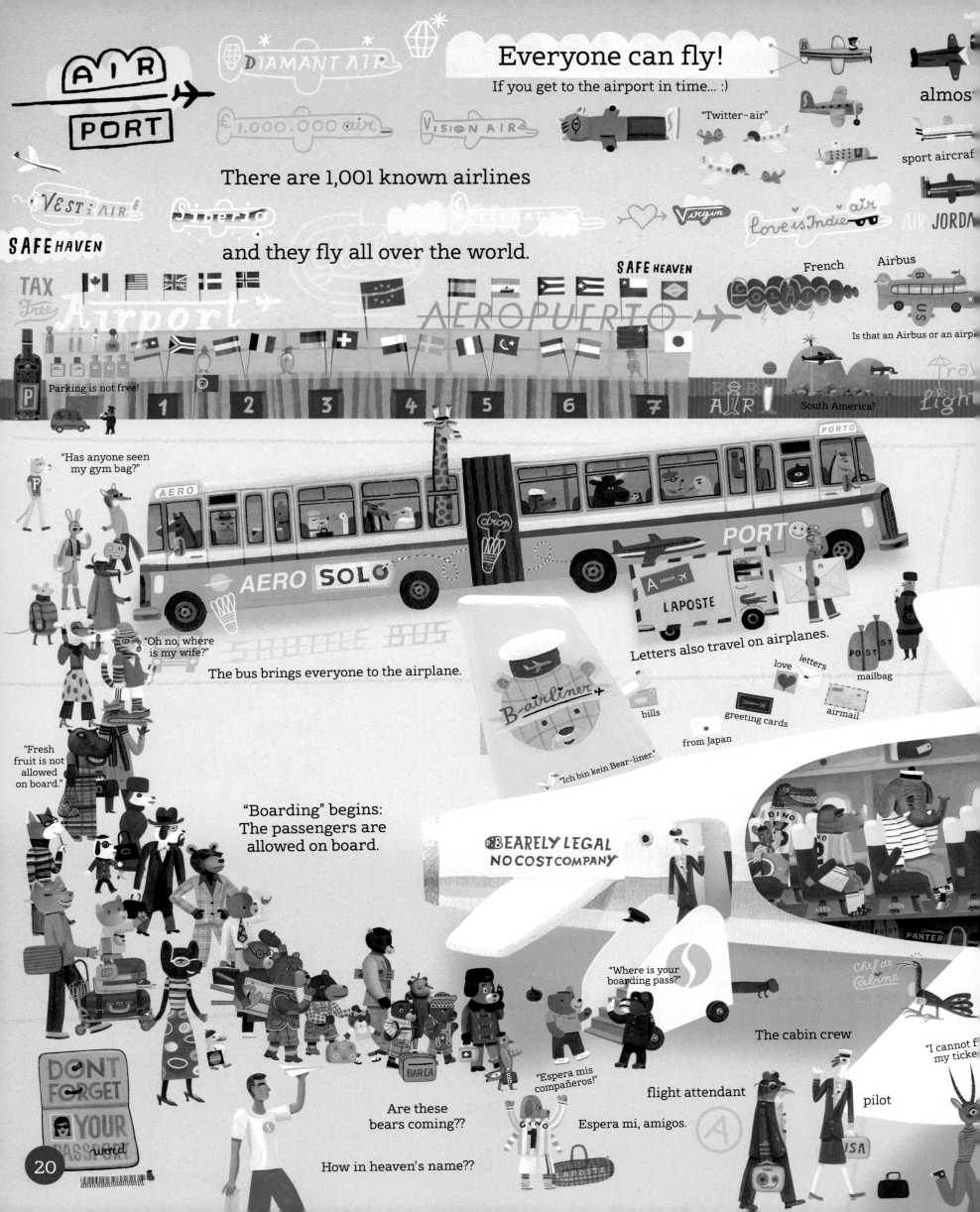

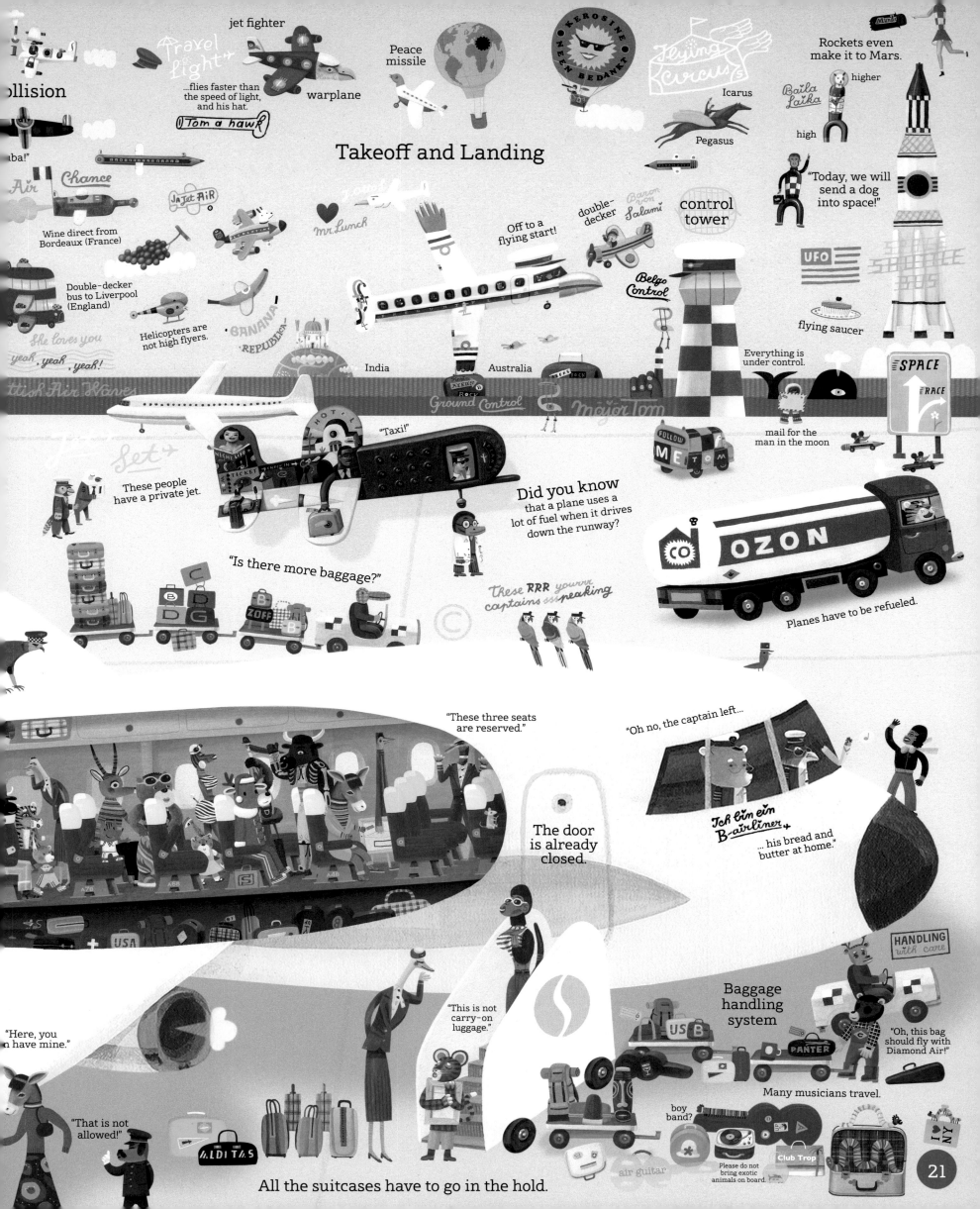

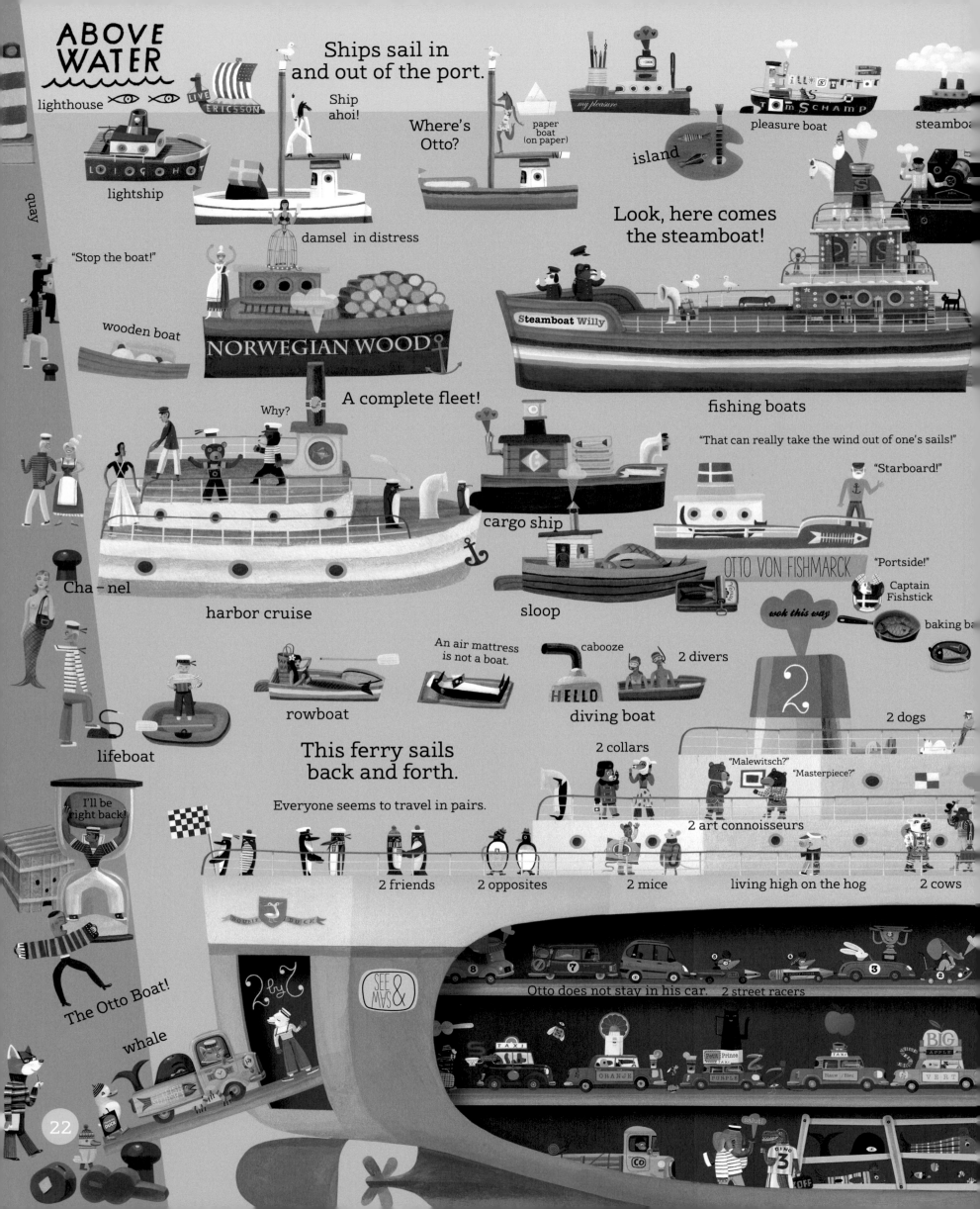

ABOVE WATER

lighthouse

LIVE ERICSSON

Ships sail in and out of the port.

Ship ahoi!

Where's Otto?

paper boat (on paper)

island

my pleasure

pleasure boat

TOM SCHAMP

steamboat

lightship

quay

damsel in distress

Look, here comes the steamboat!

"Stop the boat!"

wooden boat

NORWEGIAN WOOD

Steamboat Willy

fishing boats

A complete fleet!

Why?

"That can really take the wind out of one's sails!"

"Starboard!"

cargo ship

OTTO VON FISHMARCK

"Portside!"

Captain Fishstick

wok this way

baking ba

Cha – nel

harbor cruise

sloop

An air mattress is not a boat.

cabooze

2 divers

2 dogs

rowboat

diving boat

HELLO

lifeboat

This ferry sails back and forth.

2 collars

"Malewitsch?"

"Masterpiece?"

I'll be right back!

Everyone seems to travel in pairs.

2 art connoisseurs

2 friends

2 opposites

2 mice

living high on the hog

2 cows

DOUBLE DUCK

The Otto Boat!

2 by 7

SEE & SAW

Otto does not stay in his car.

2 street racers

TAXI

Petit Prince

TAXI

BIG APPLE

whale

ORANJE

PURPLE

Blauw / Bleu

VERT

22

CO

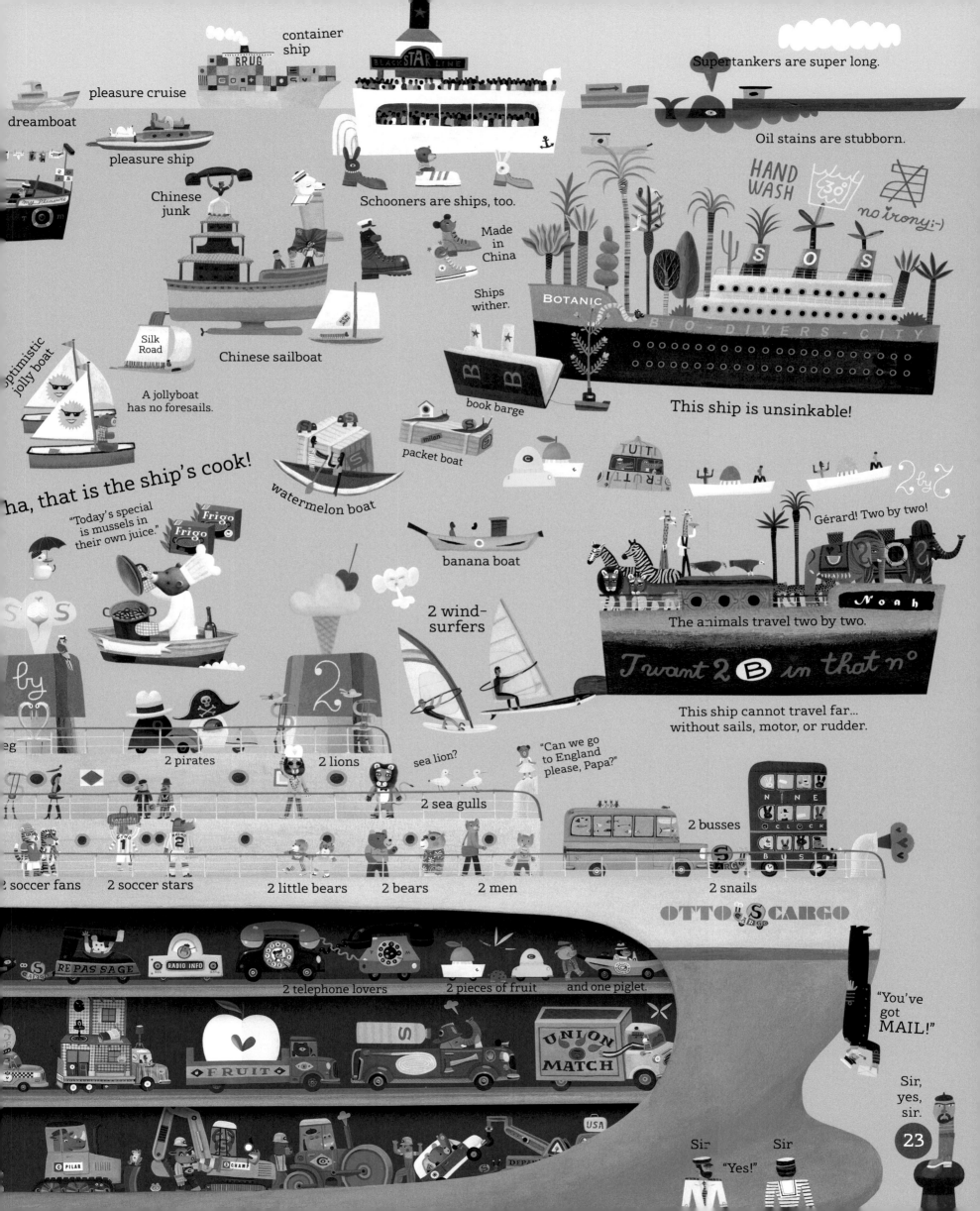

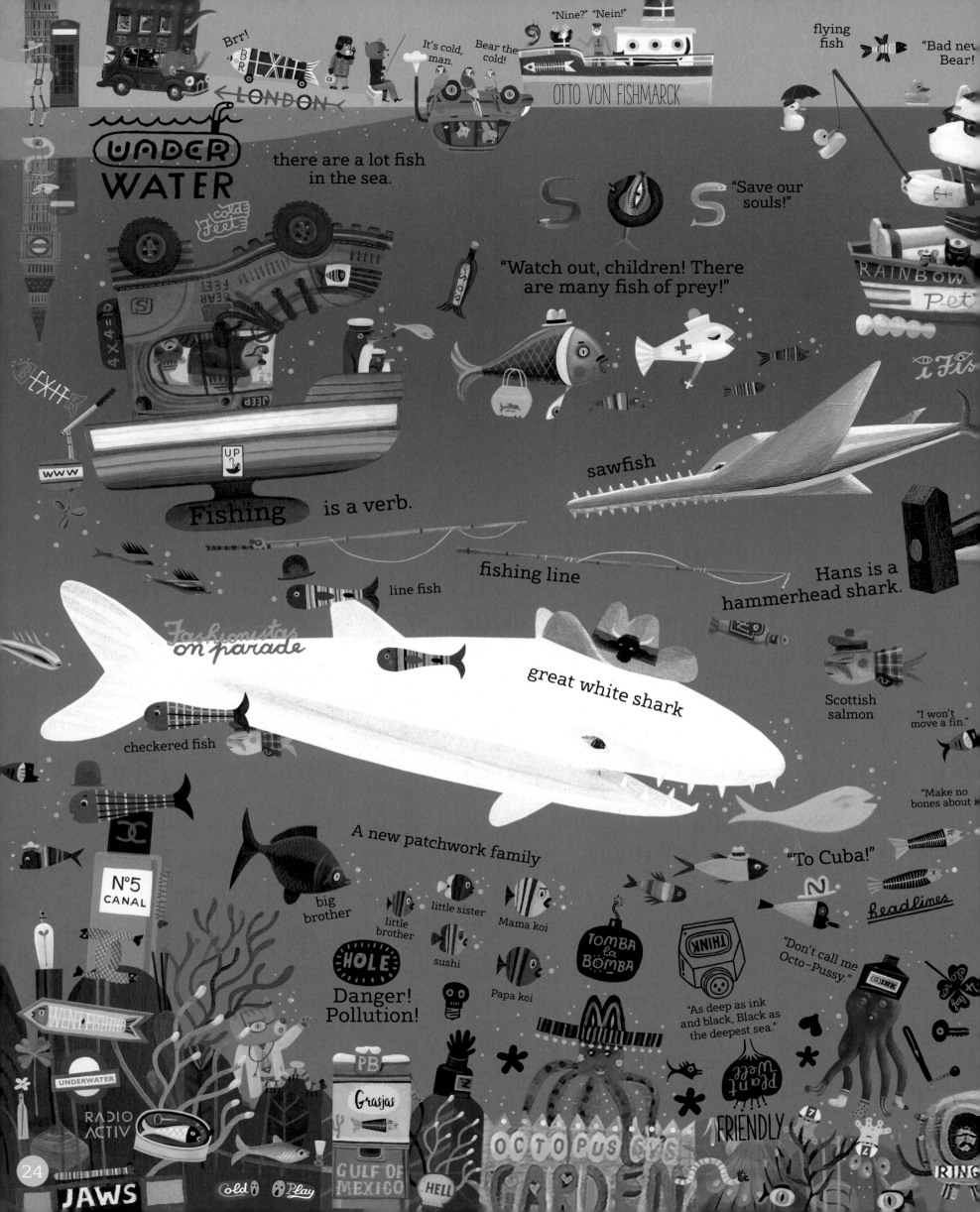

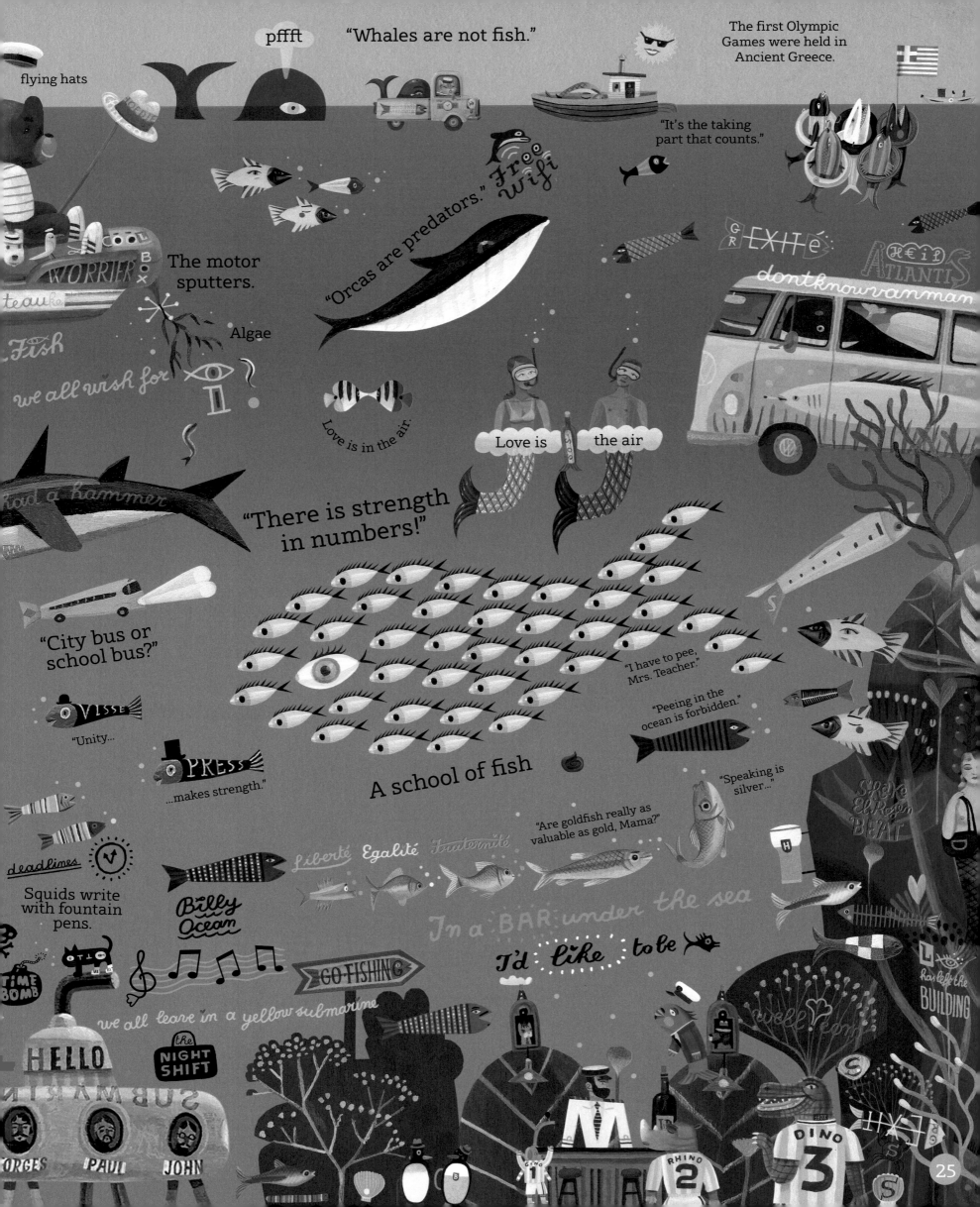

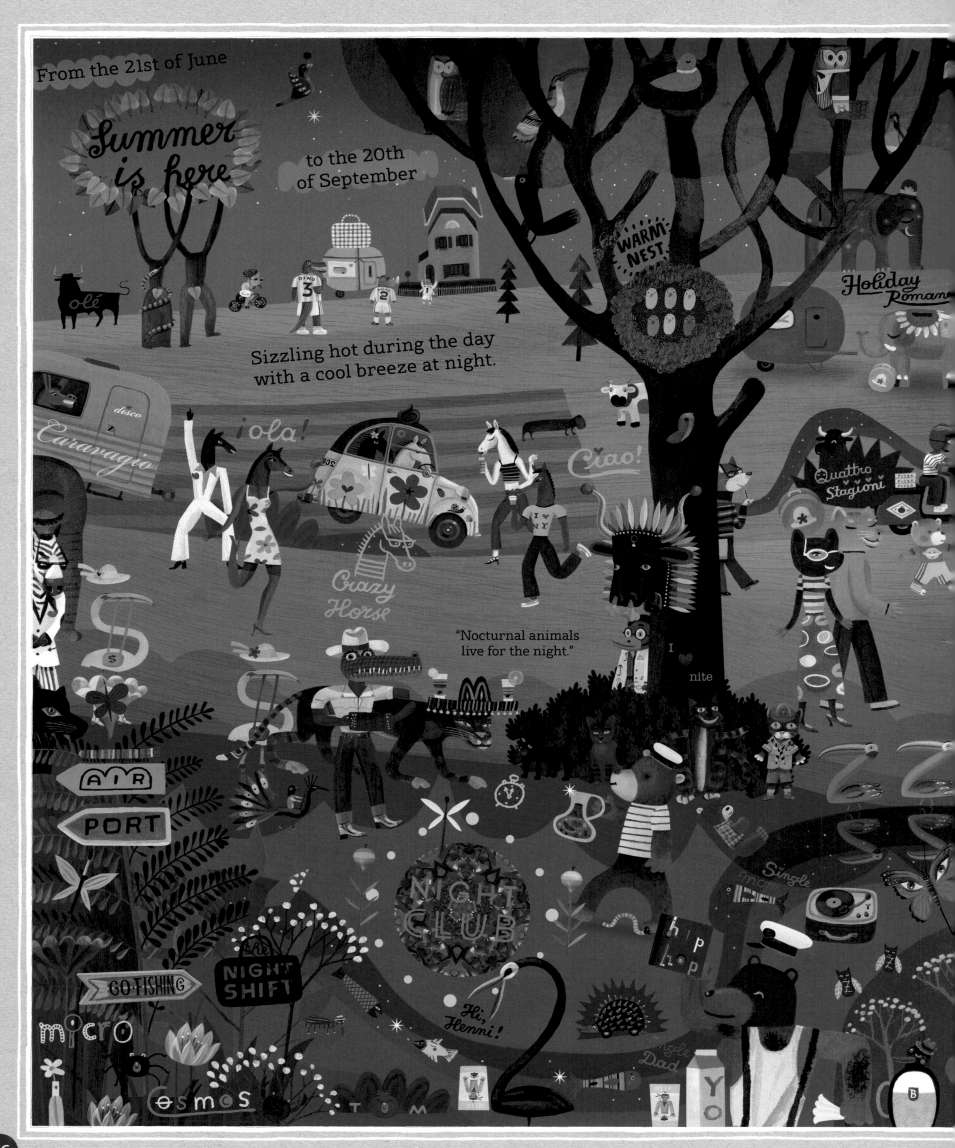

From the 21st of June

Summer is here

to the 20th of September

Sizzling hot during the day with a cool breeze at night.

"Nocturnal animals live for the night."

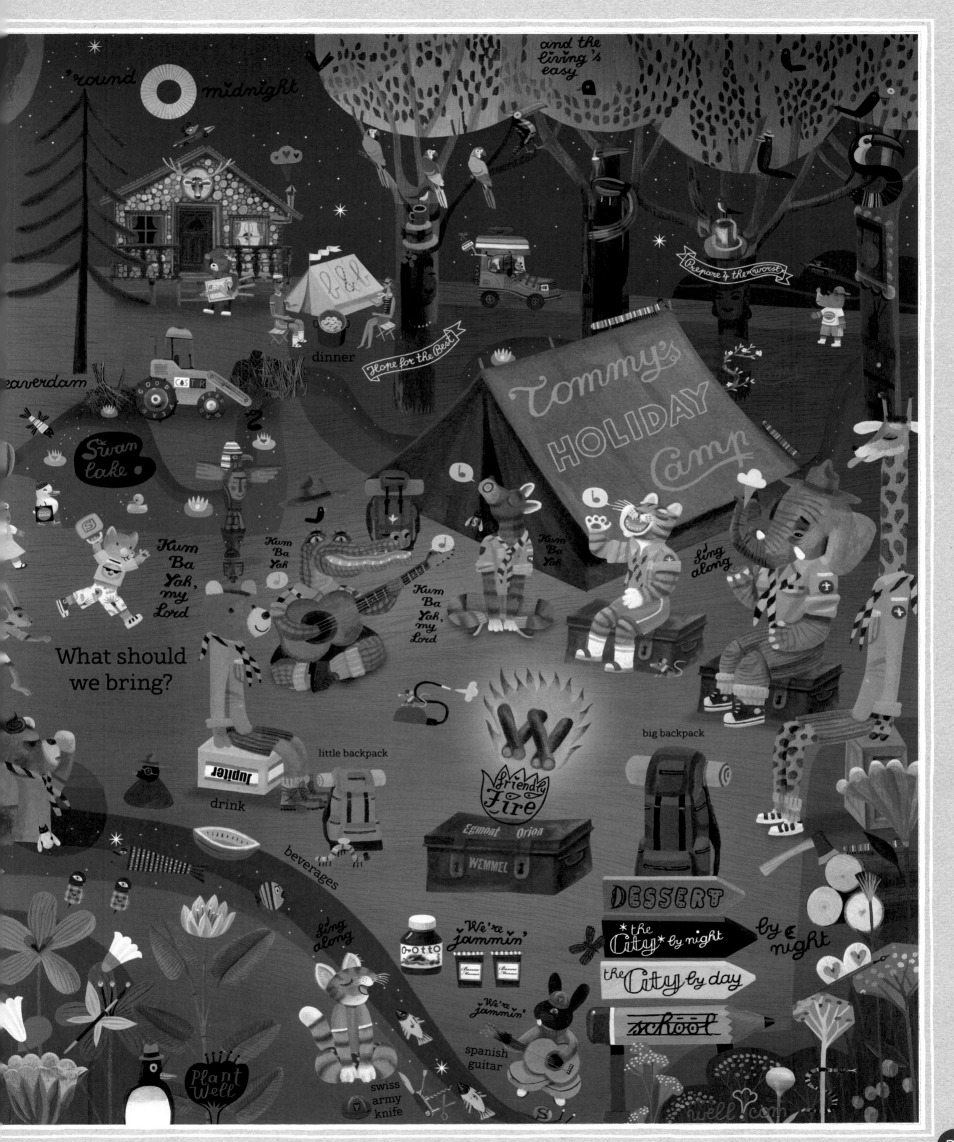

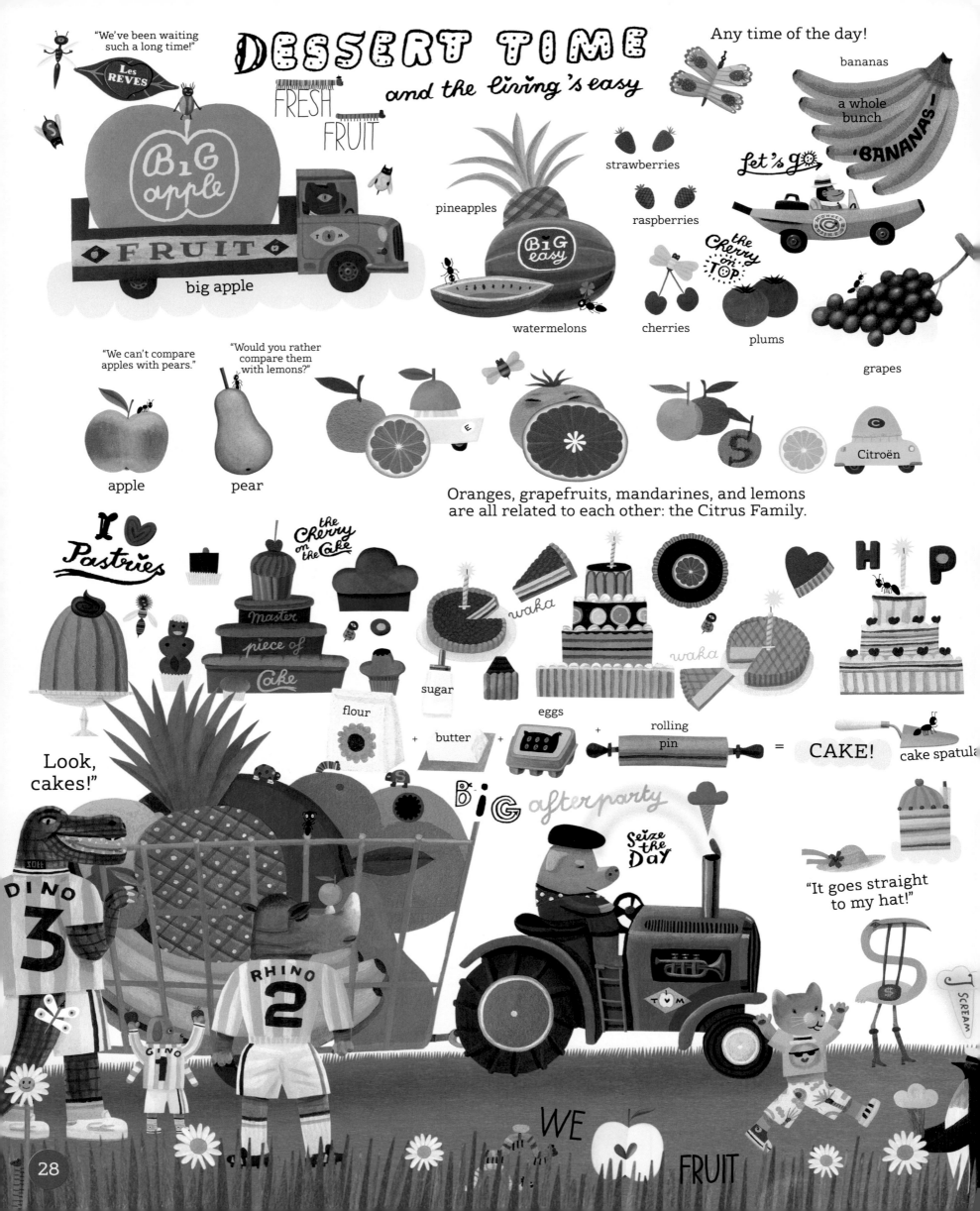

DESSERT TIME
and the living's easy

"We've been waiting such a long time!"

Les REVES

Any time of the day!

bananas

a whole bunch

BANANAS

Let's go

FRESH FRUIT

B1G apple

FRUIT

big apple

pineapples

B1G easy

strawberries

raspberries

the Cherry on TOP

cherries

plums

watermelons

grapes

"We can't compare apples with pears."

"Would you rather compare them with lemons?"

apple

pear

E

S

Citroën

Oranges, grapefruits, mandarines, and lemons are all related to each other: the Citrus Family.

I ♥ Pastries

the Cherry on the Cake

master piece of Cake

waka

waka

H P

sugar

flour + butter + eggs + rolling pin = CAKE!

cake spatula

Look, cakes!"

B1G afterparty

Seize the Day

"It goes straight to my hat!"

DINO 3

RHINO 2

GINO 1

$

$

I SCREAM

WE ♥ FRUIT

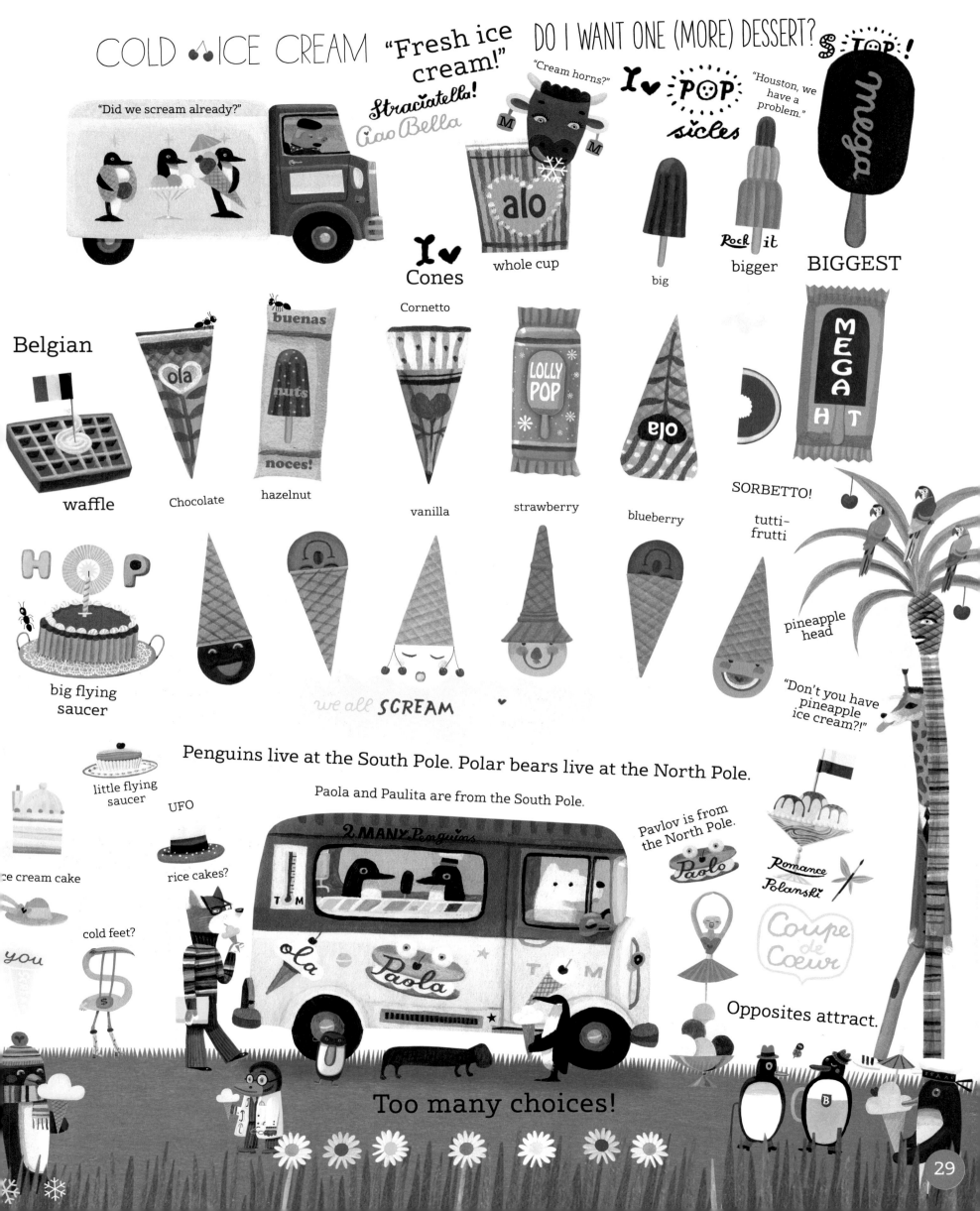

COLD ICE CREAM

"Fresh ice cream!"

Straciatella!

Ciao Bella

"Did we scream already?"

DO I WANT ONE (MORE) DESSERT?

"Cream horns?"

I ♥ POPsicles

"Houston, we have a problem."

STOP!

mega

I ♥ Cones

whole cup — alo

big

Rock it — bigger

BIGGEST

Belgian

waffle

Chocolate — ola

hazelnut — buenas nuts noces!

Cornetto

vanilla

strawberry — LOLLY POP

blueberry — ejo ola

SORBETTO!

tutti-frutti

MEGA HIT

big flying saucer — HOP

we all SCREAM ♥

pineapple head

"Don't you have pineapple ice cream?!"

little flying saucer

UFO

ice cream cake

rice cakes?

cold feet?

you

Penguins live at the South Pole. Polar bears live at the North Pole.

Paola and Paulita are from the South Pole.

2 MANY Penguins

ola Paola

T M — T M

Pavlov is from the North Pole.

Paolo

Romance Polanski

Coupe de Coeur

Opposites attract.

Too many choices!

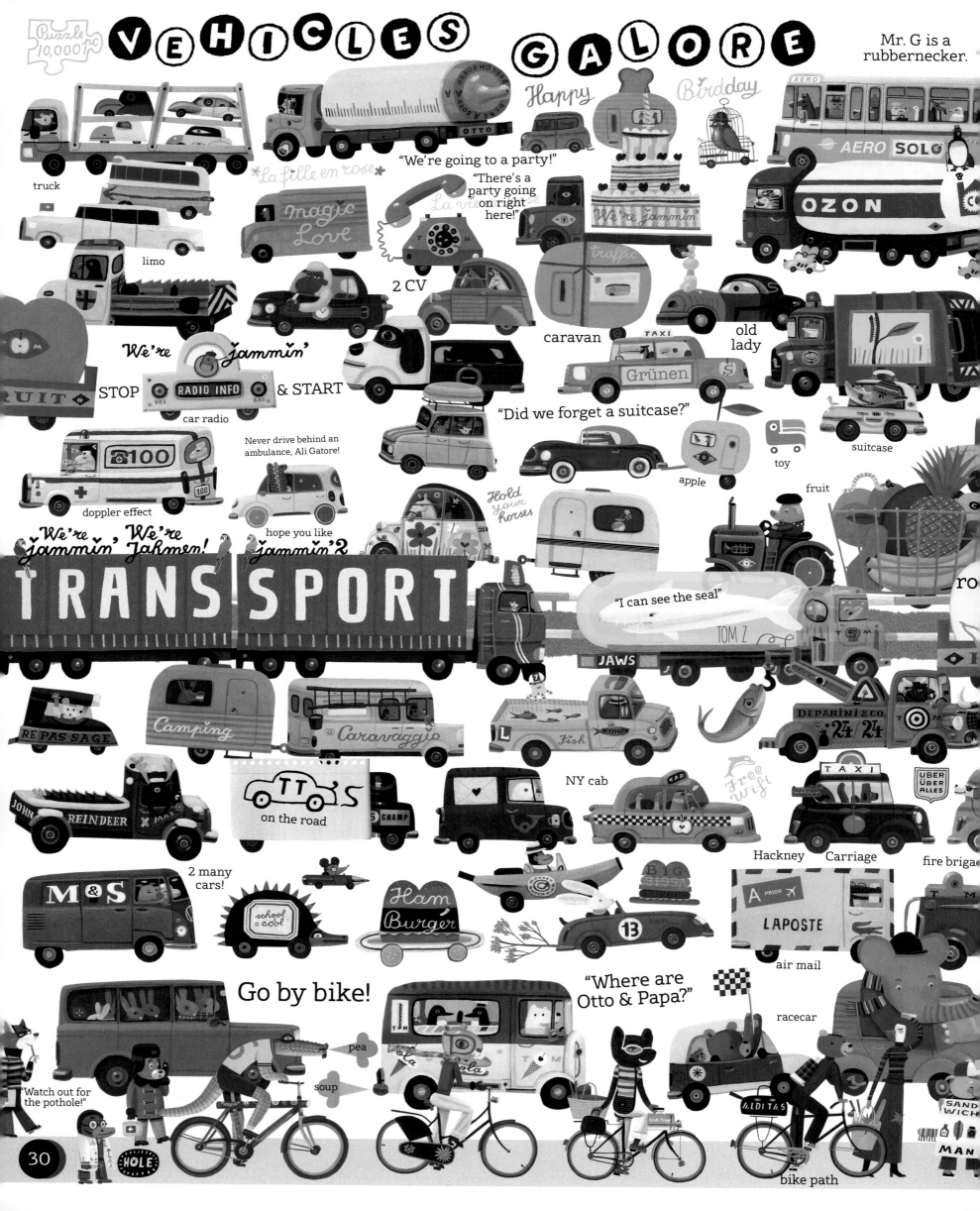

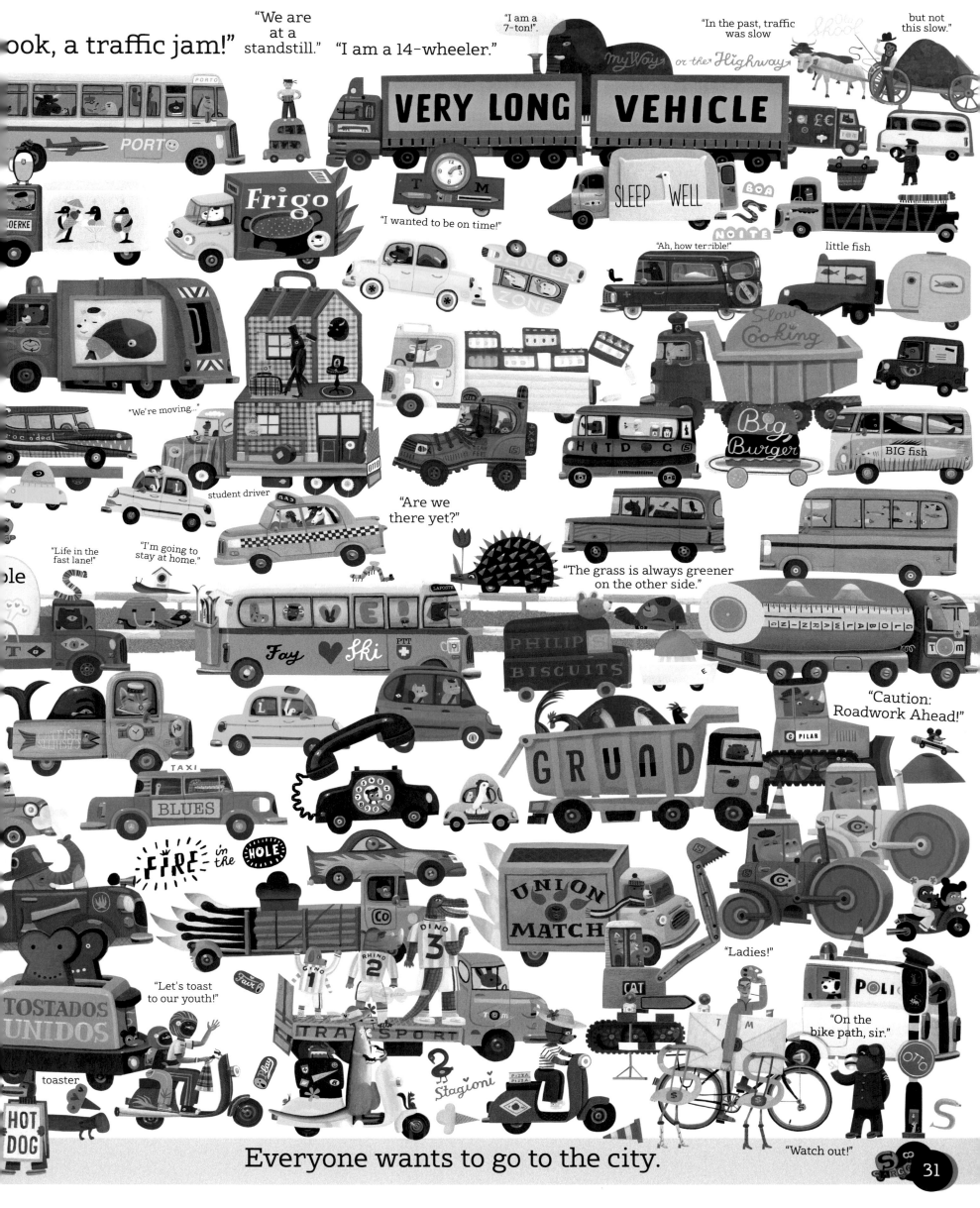

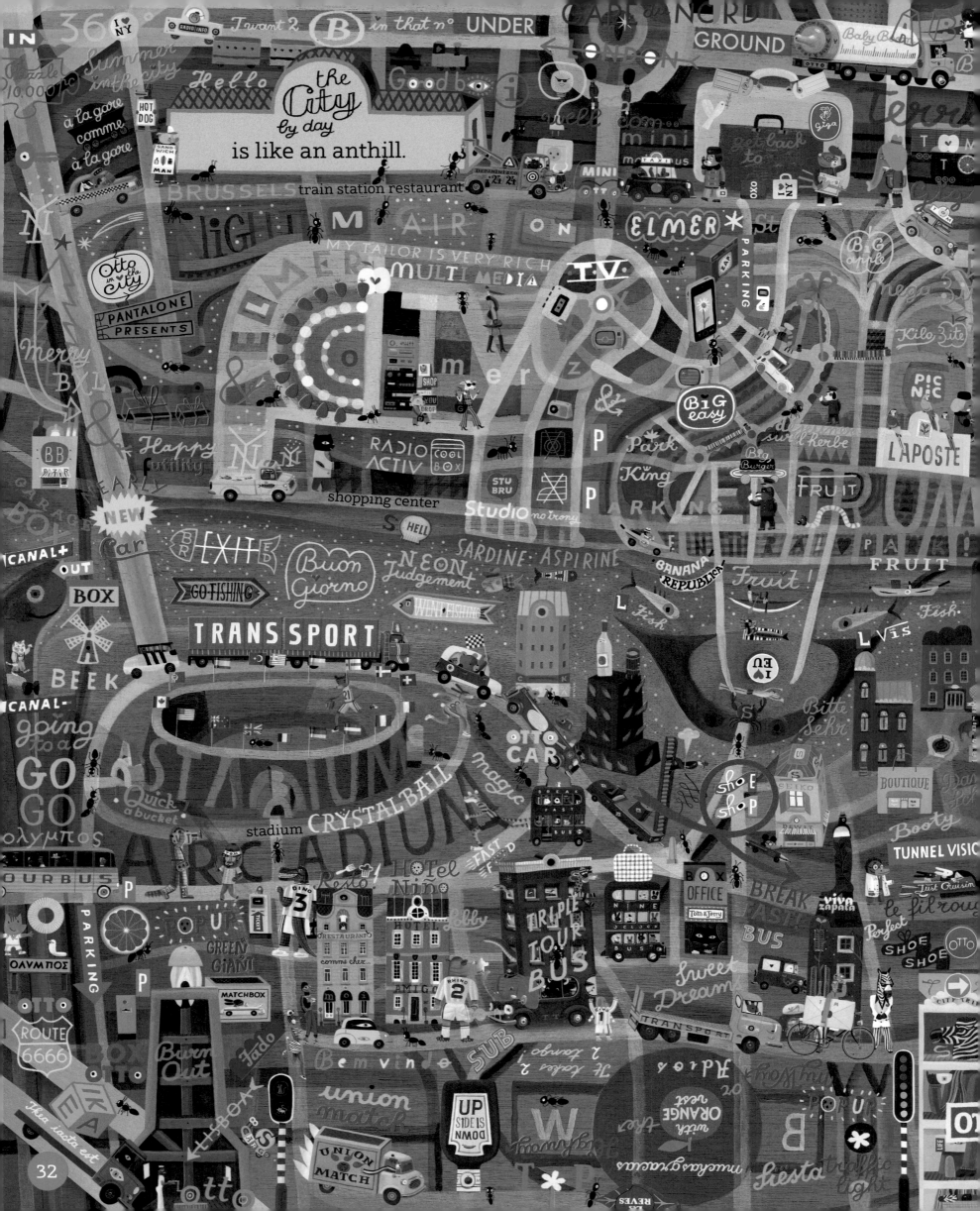

the City by day is like an anthill.

train station restaurant

shopping center

stadium

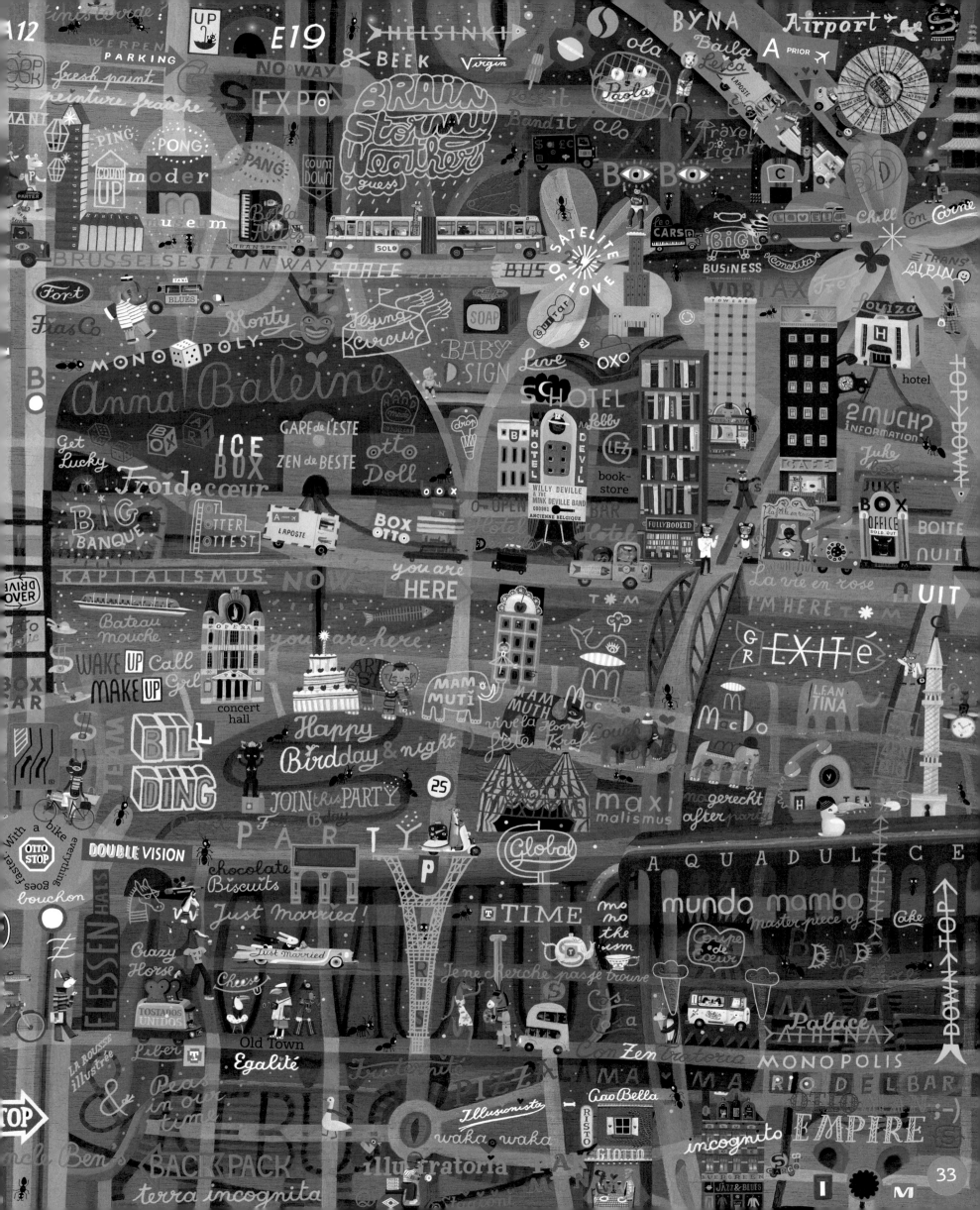

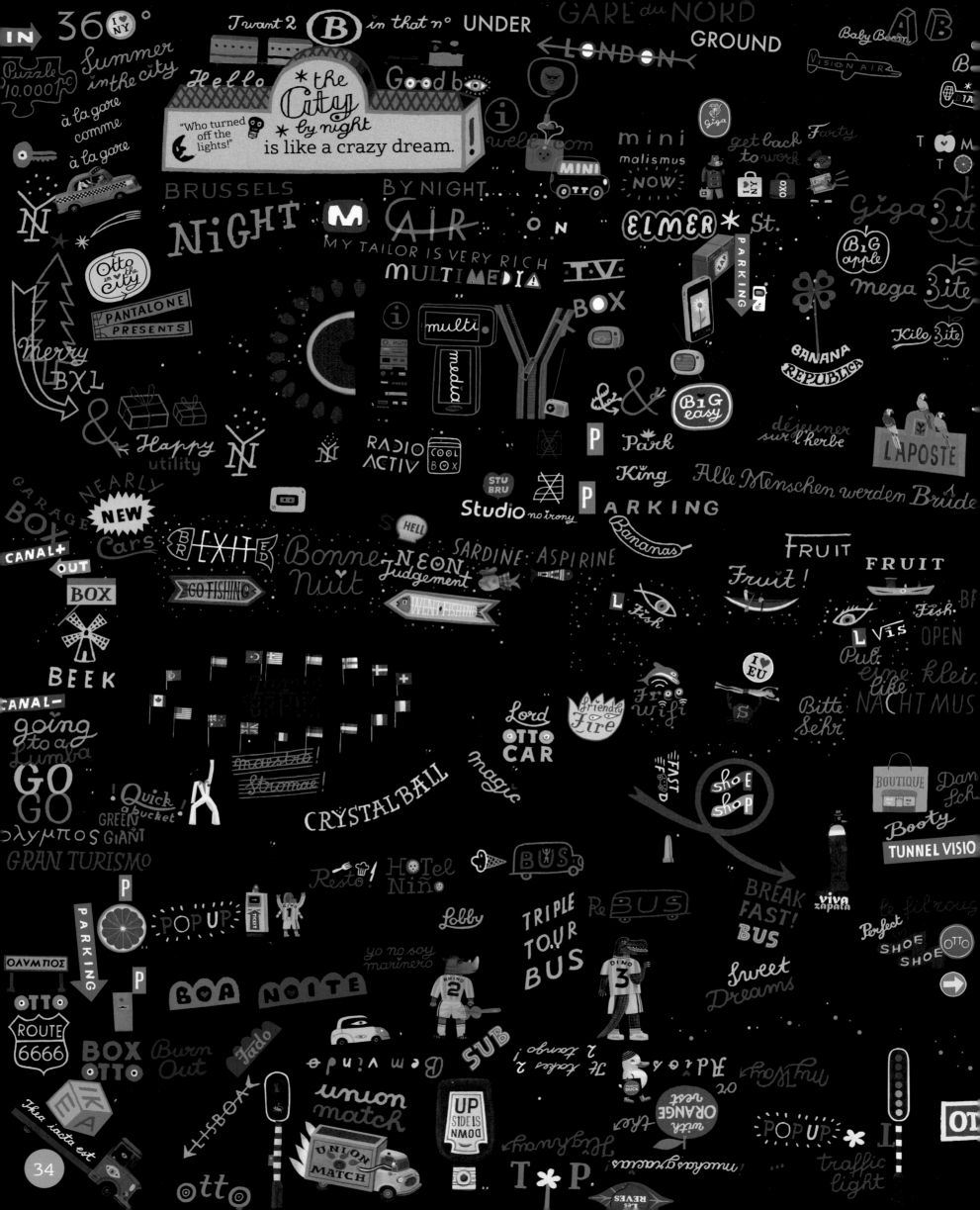

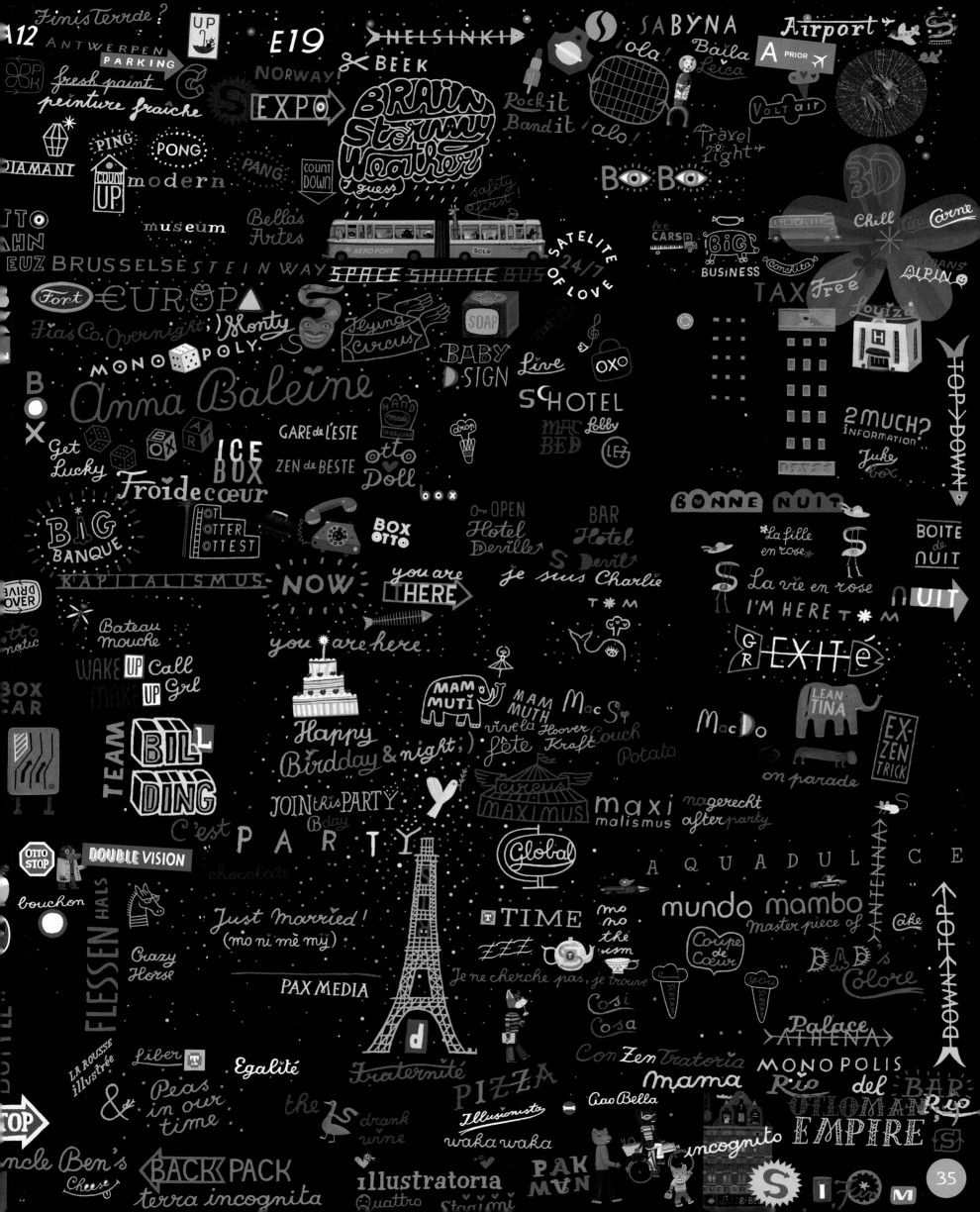

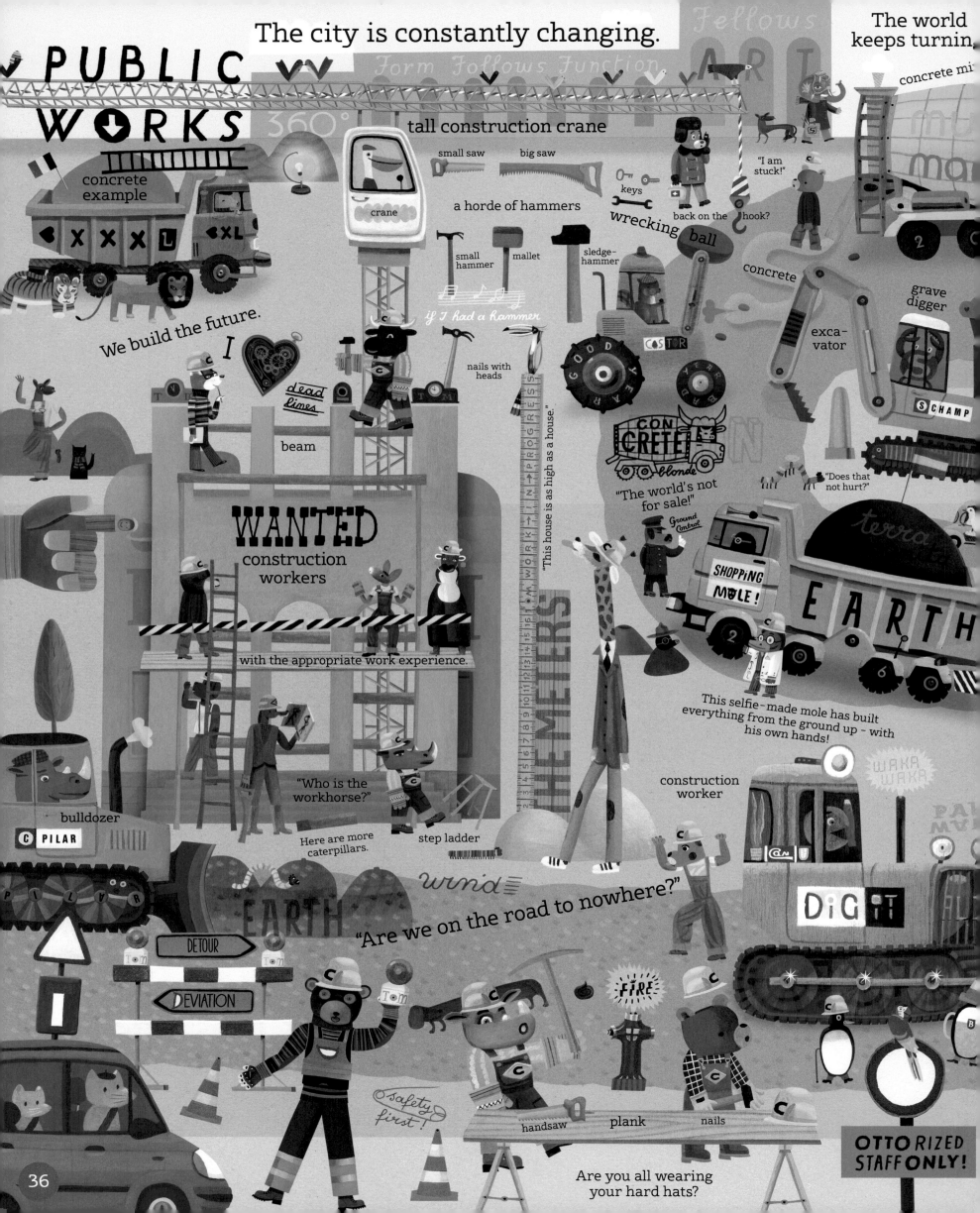

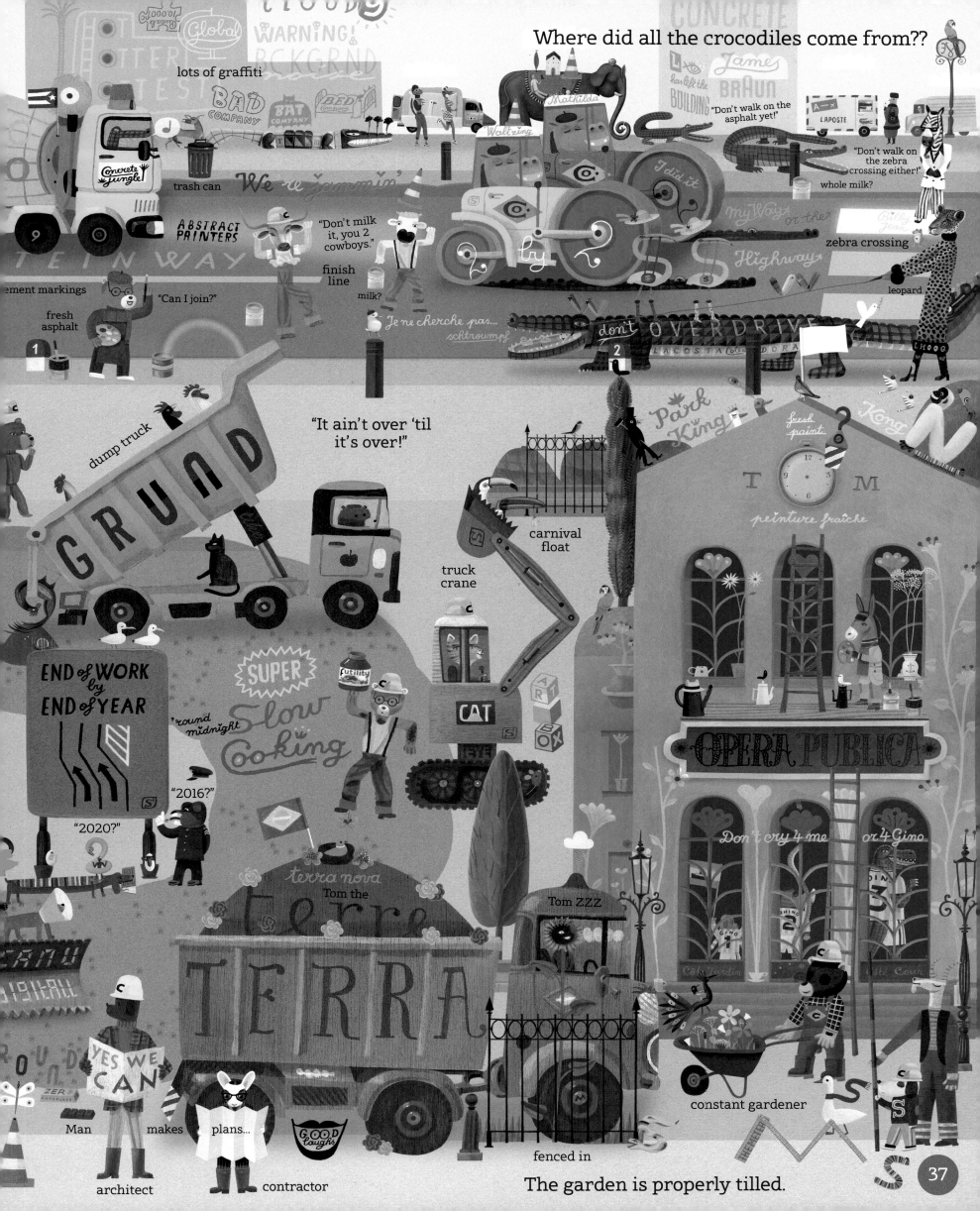

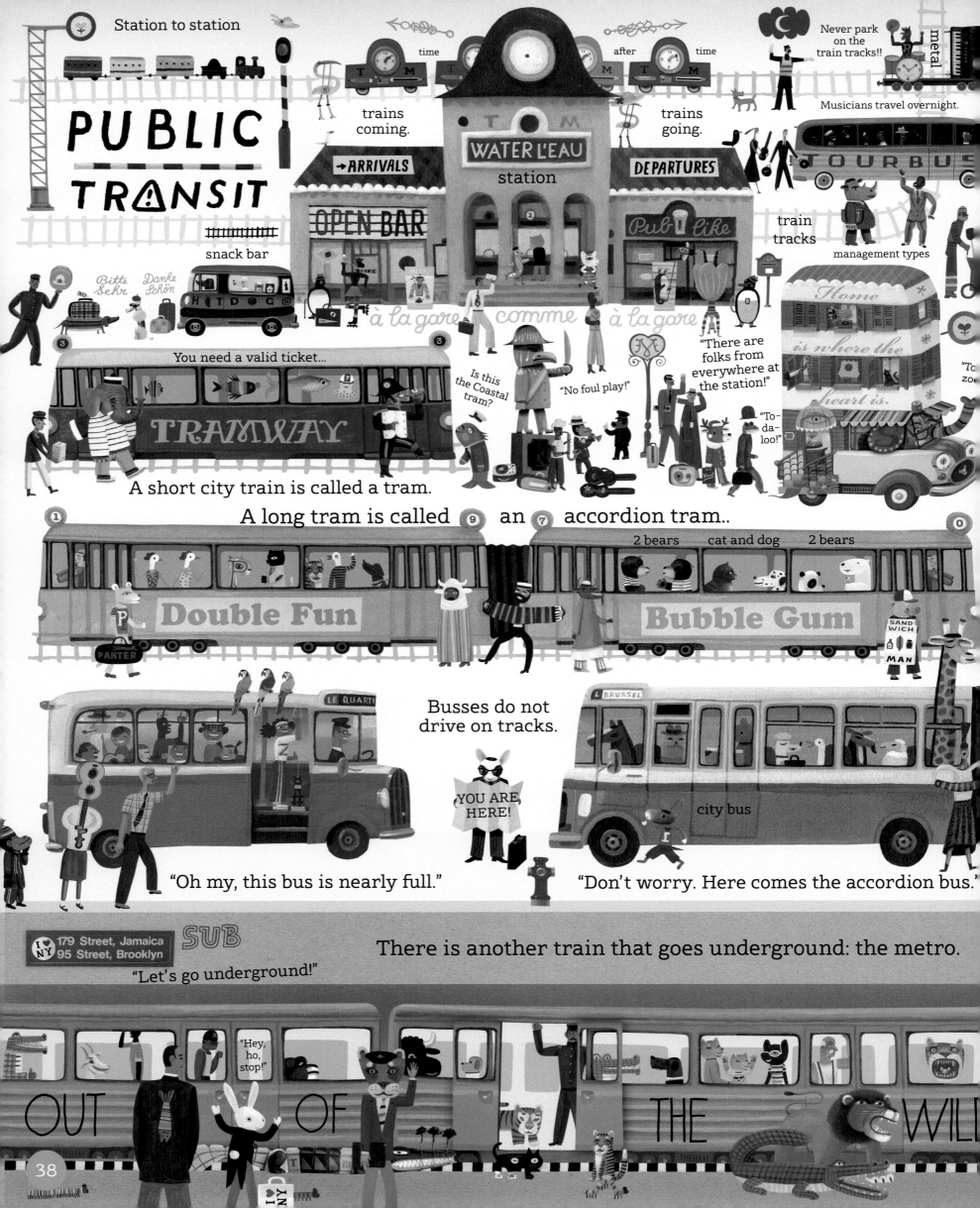

Station to station

PUBLIC
TRANSIT

Never park on the train tracks!!

Musicians travel overnight.

time trains coming. after time trains going.

WATER L'EAU
station

→ ARRIVALS   DEPARTURES

TOURBUS

OPEN BAR   Pub like

snack bar

train tracks

management types

Bitte Sehr   Danke Schön

HOT DOGS

à la gare   comme   à la gare

Home is where the heart is.

You need a valid ticket...

Is this the Coastal tram?

"No foul play!"

"There are folks from everywhere at the station!"

"To-da-loo!"

TRAMWAY

A short city train is called a tram.

A long tram is called an accordion tram..

2 bears   cat and dog   2 bears

Double Fun   Bubble Gum

PANTER

SAND WICH

MAN

LE QUARTI

Busses do not drive on tracks.

YOU ARE HERE!

L BRUSSEL

city bus

"Oh my, this bus is nearly full."

"Don't worry. Here comes the accordion bus."

179 Street, Jamaica
95 Street, Brooklyn

SUB   There is another train that goes underground: the metro.

"Let's go underground!"

"Hey, ho, stop!"

OUT   OF   THE   WIL

Freight trains often travel overnight. They are very long and do not transport people. And, the heavier their cargo, the more noise they make.

conductor

electric locomotive

train car

night train

overnight train

WAGONS LITS

sleep

well

"I'll have gone 500 miles when the day is done."

"We will be there in the early morning."

"I am already dreaming of winter vocation."

BEST SKI

day train

SWISS

"Do you have enough coal on board, Bernhard?"

steam train

BUS

tour-bus

Re BUS

"Papa?"

"Watch out: in England their right is our left!"

"That's right!"

"You're left!"

VERY HIGH HOUSE

London has double-decker busses.

"check"

"double check"

"Wait, do you know when we change?"

BREAK FAST BUS

double

triple-decker

NINE O CLOCK BUS

YOU DROP

quadruple-decker

merry Christmas Happy NEW year

VELVET UNDERGROUND

CAFE

SHOP UNTIL YOU DROP

final stop

The metro system is also called U-Bahn, the tube, or the subway.

subway operator

tax free zone

ON bus ker THE ROAD

"Don't stand on or near the tracks!"

escalator

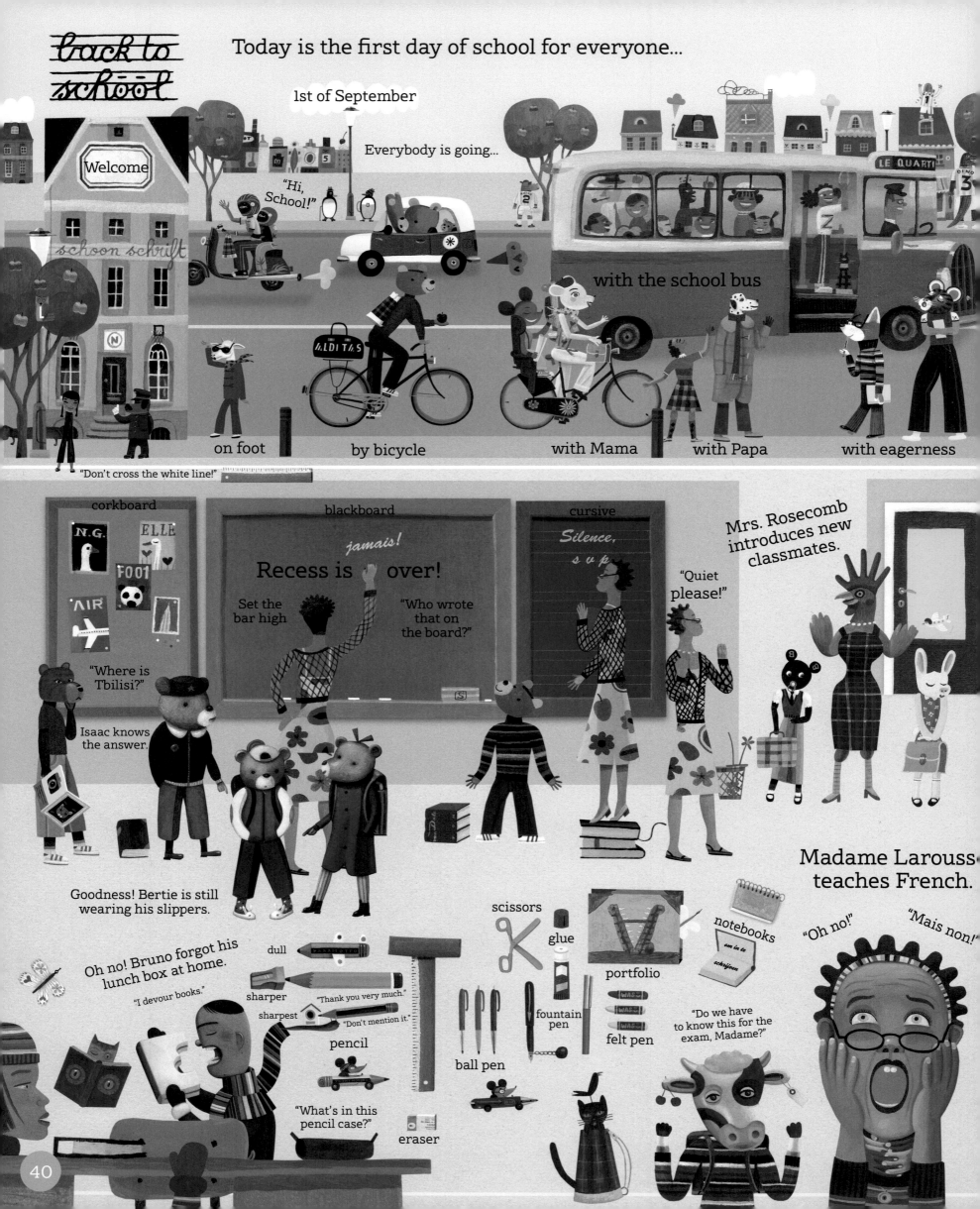

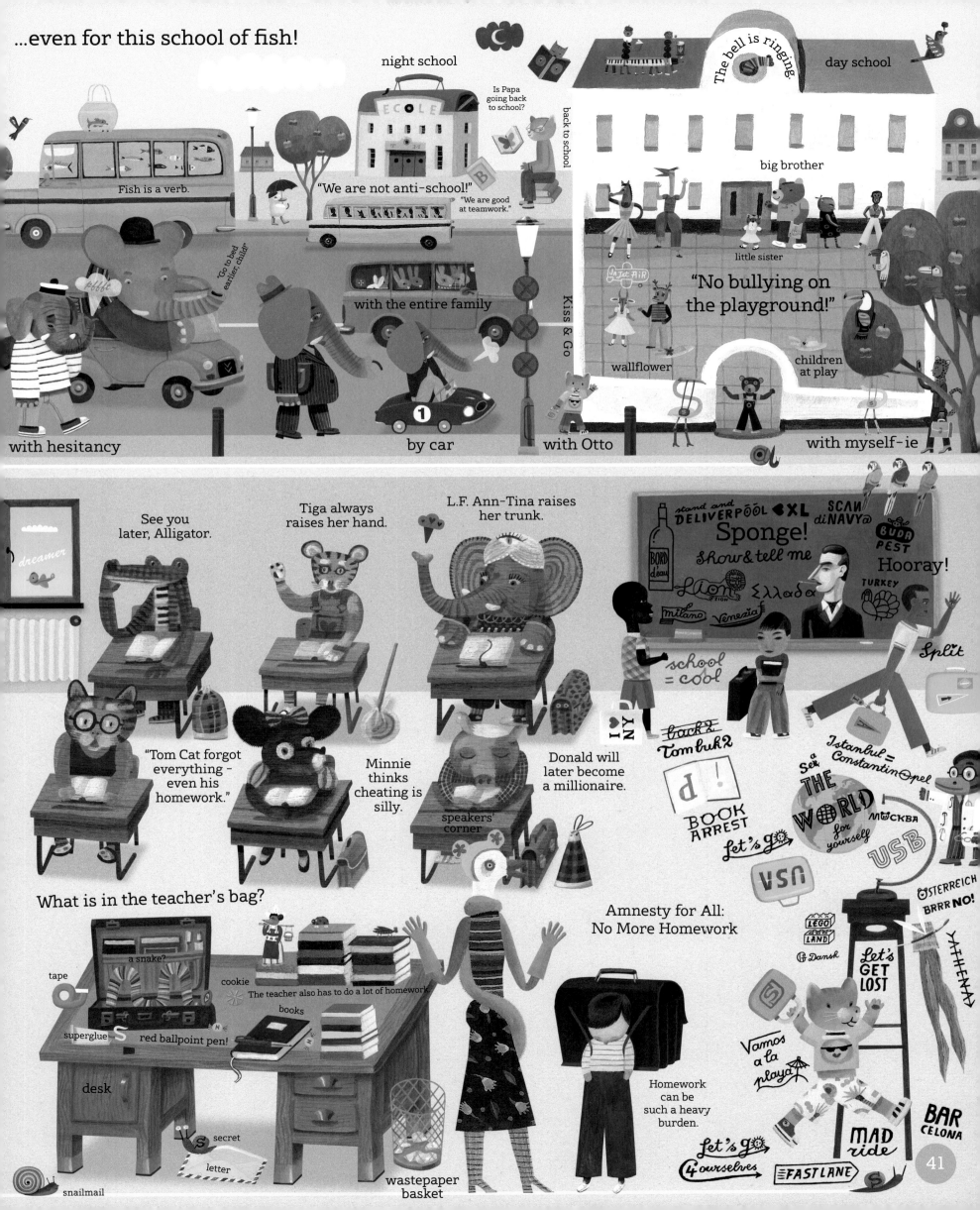

...even for this school of fish!

Fish is a verb.

with hesitancy

night school

Is Papa going back to school?

back to school

"We are not anti-school!"

"We are good at teamwork."

with the entire family

Kiss & Go

by car

"Go to bed earlier, child"

with Otto

The bell is ringing.

day school

big brother

little sister

"No bullying on the playground!"

wallflower

children at play

with myself-ie

dreamer

See you later, Alligator.

Tiga always raises her hand.

L.F. Ann-Tina raises her trunk.

stand and DELIVERPÖÖL ◆XL
SCAN diNAVY@
Sponge!
BORDeaux
Show & tell me
BUDA PEST
Lion
Ελλάδα
TURKEY
Hooray!
Milano Venezia

"Tom Cat forgot everything – even his homework."

Minnie thinks cheating is silly.

Donald will later become a millionaire.

speakers' corner

school = cool

I ♥ NY

back 2 Tombuk2

d !

BOOK ARREST

Let's go

USA

See THE WORLD for yourself

МОСКВА

Istanbul = ConstantinOpel

USB

What is in the teacher's bag?

tape

a snake?

superglue

red ballpoint pen!

cookie

The teacher also has to do a lot of homework.

books

desk

secret

letter

snailmail

wastepaper basket

Amnesty for All:
No More Homework

Homework can be such a heavy burden.

LEGO LAND

Danish

ÖSTERREICH
BRRR NO!

Let's GET LOST

ATHENA

Vamos a la playa

BAR CELONA

Let's go 4 ourselves

FAST LANE

MAD ride

Split

41

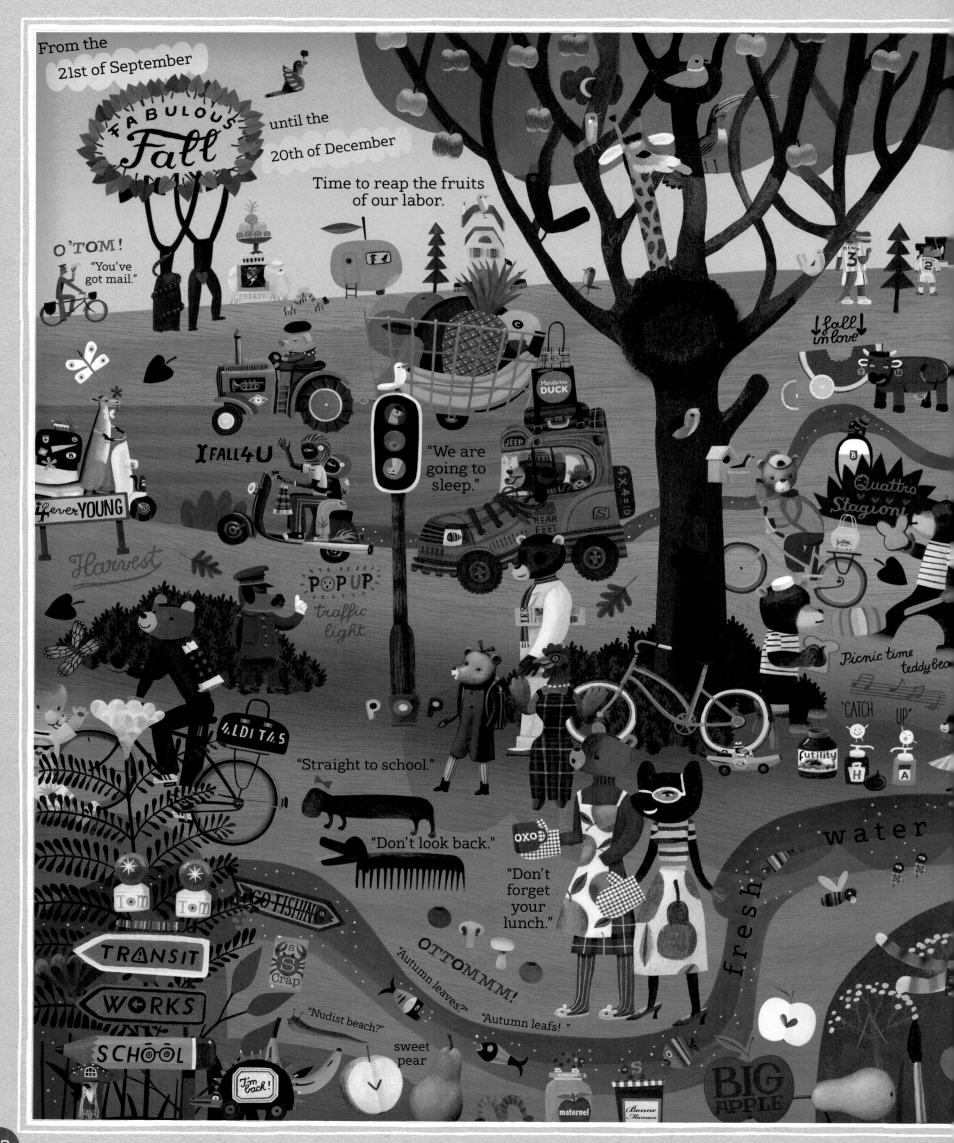

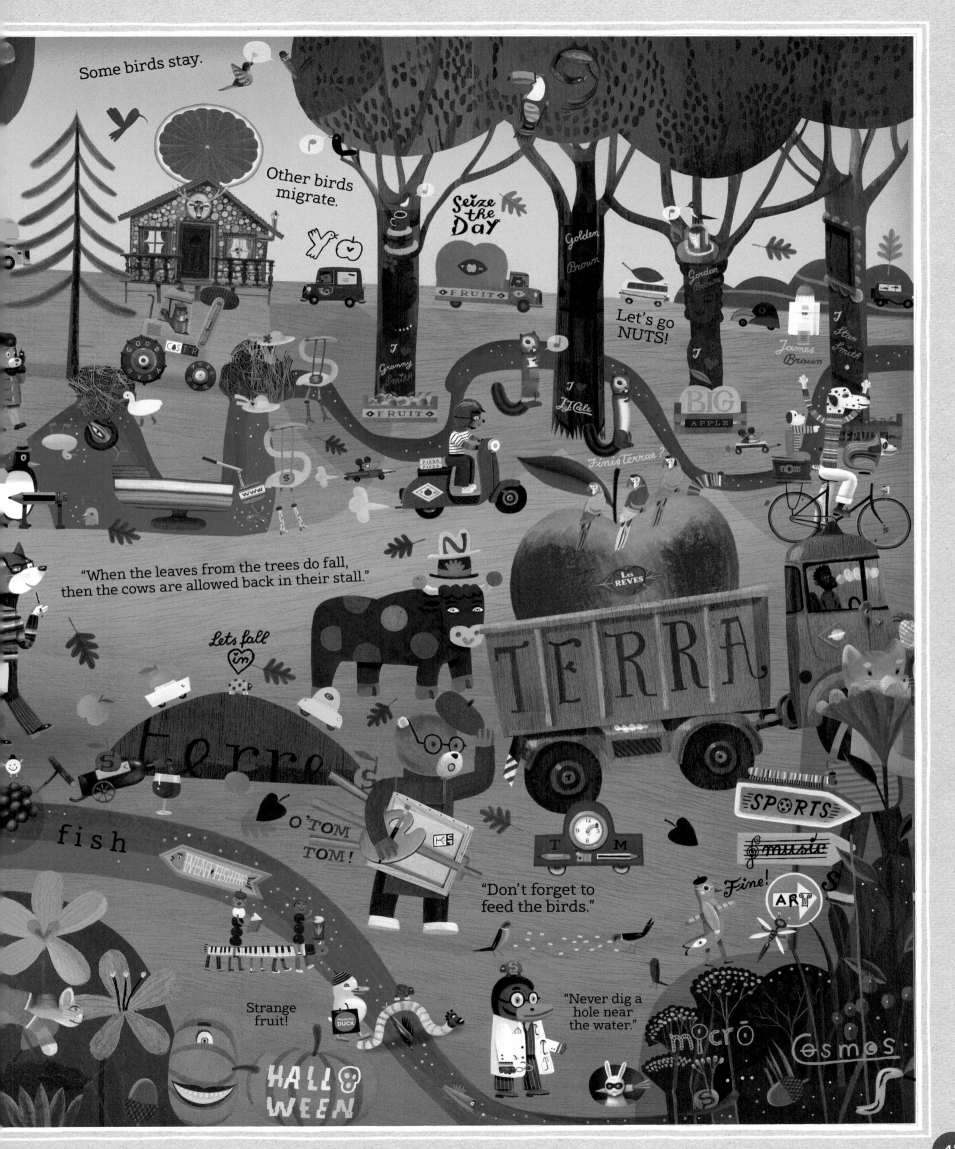

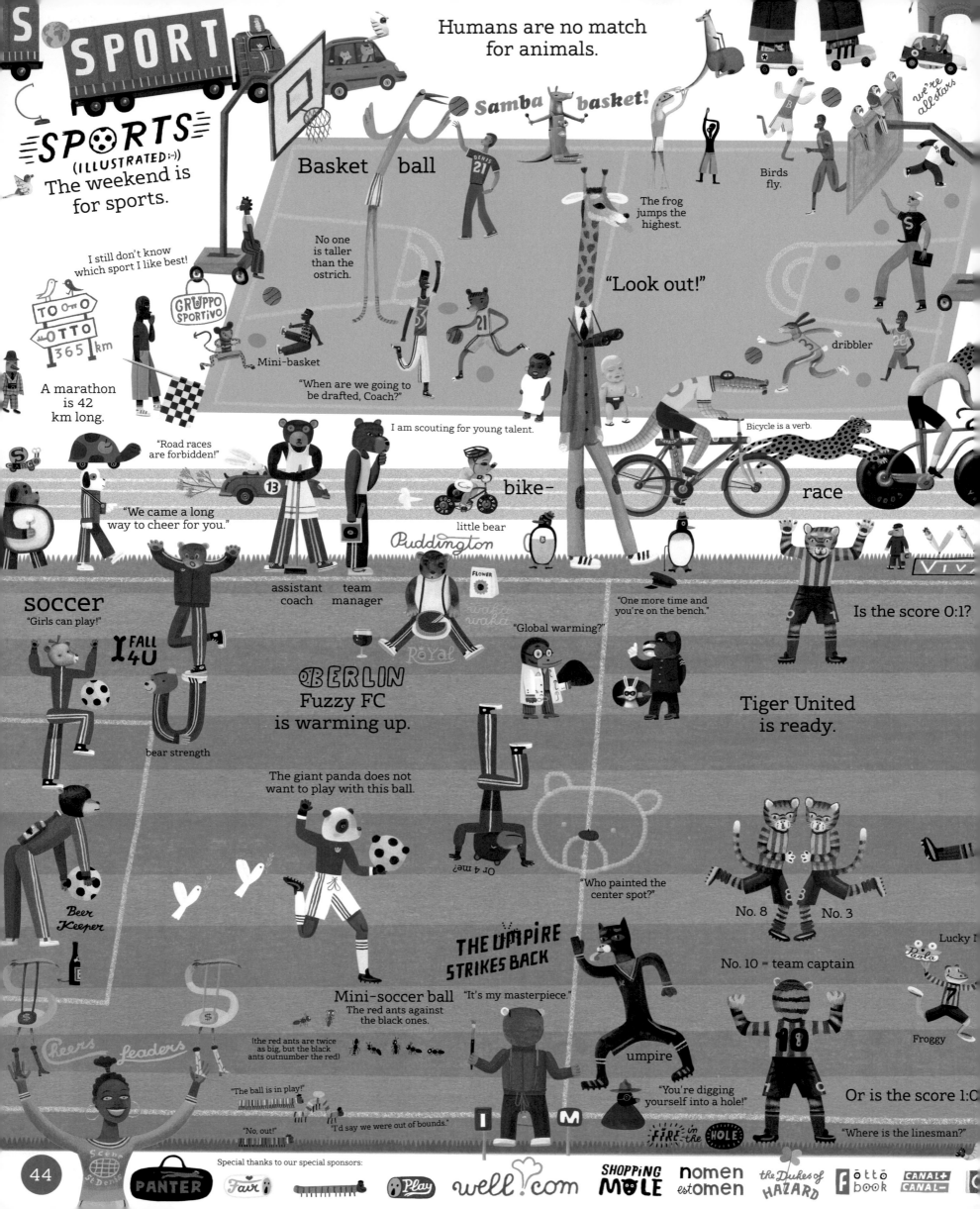

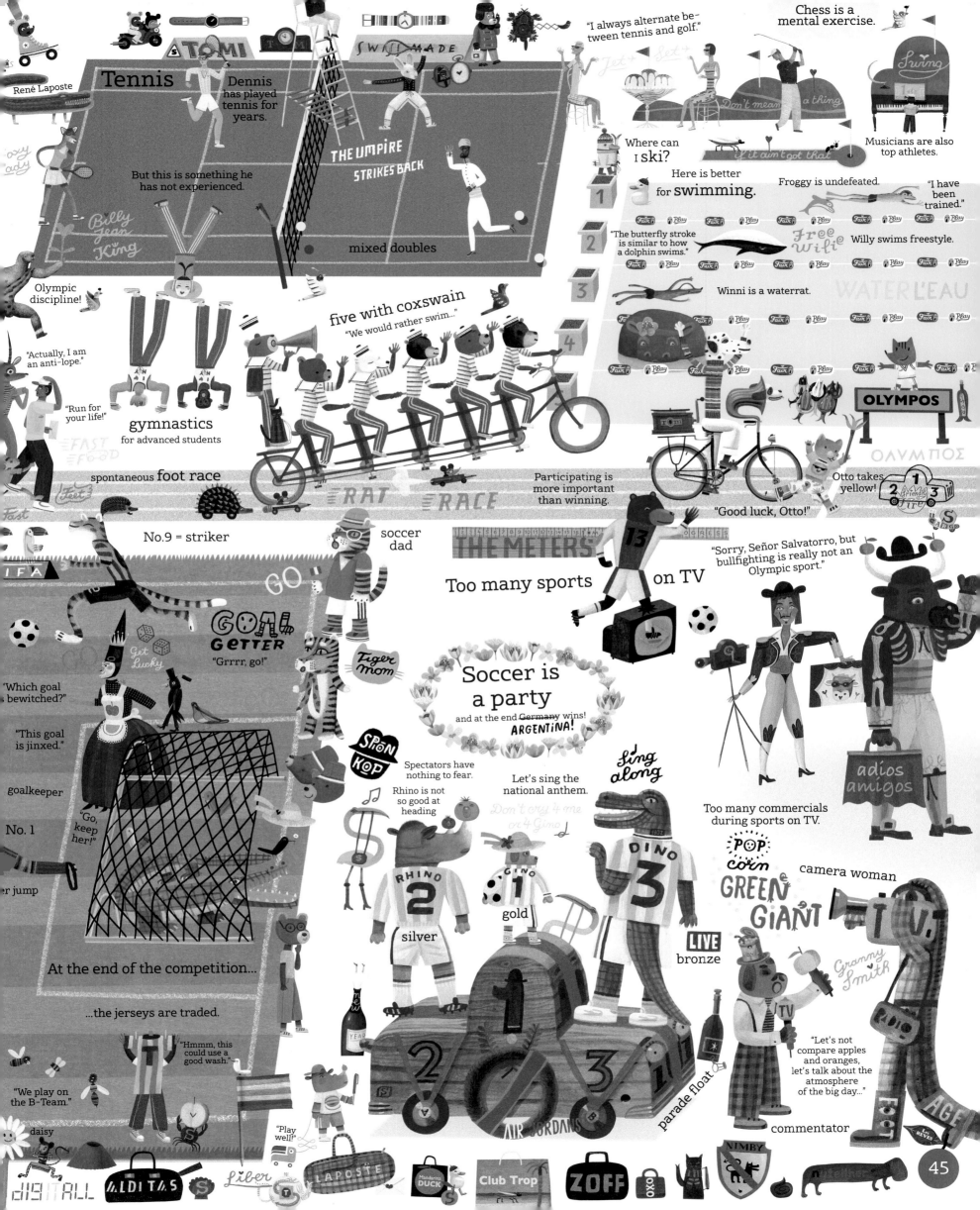

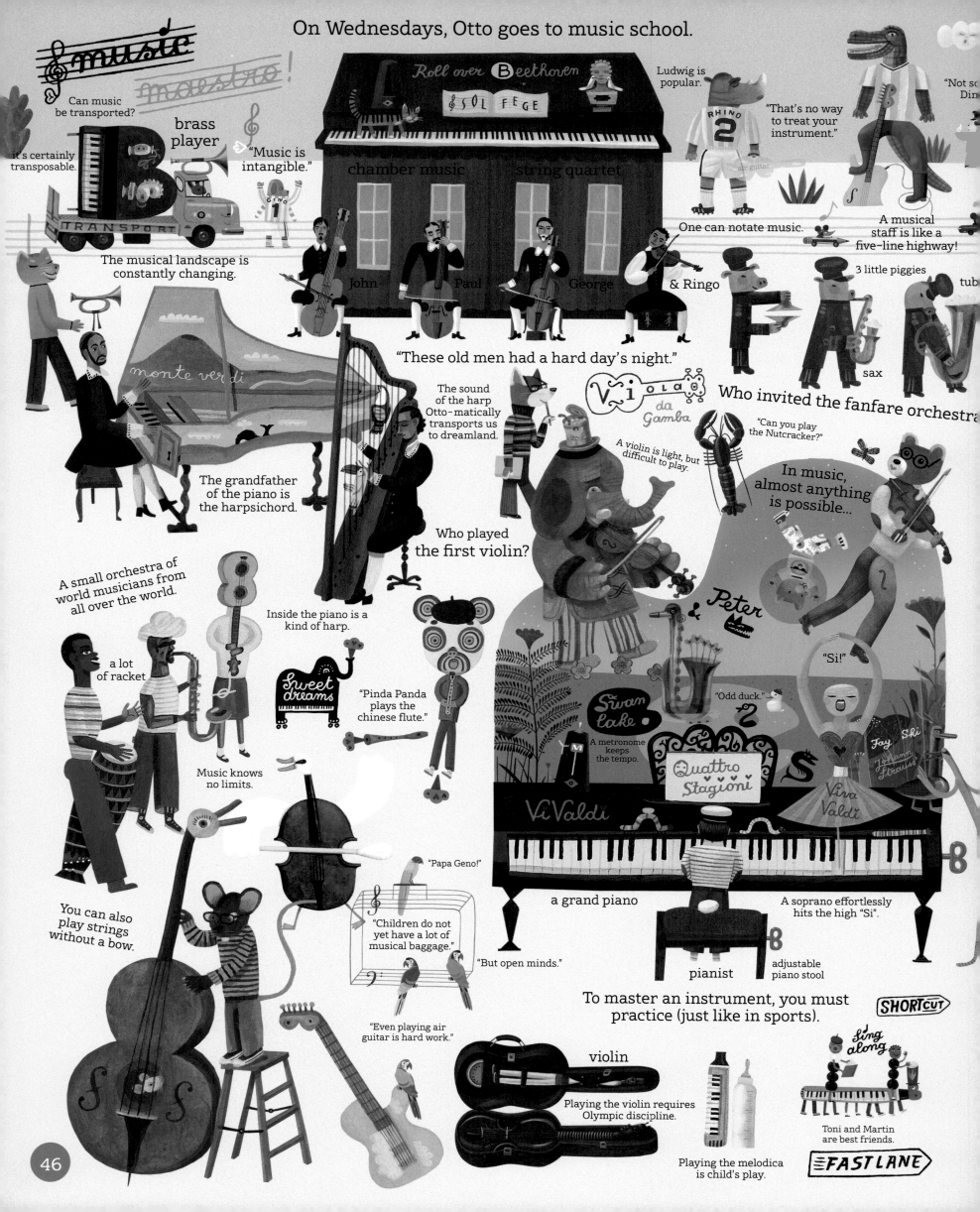

On Wednesdays, Otto goes to music school.

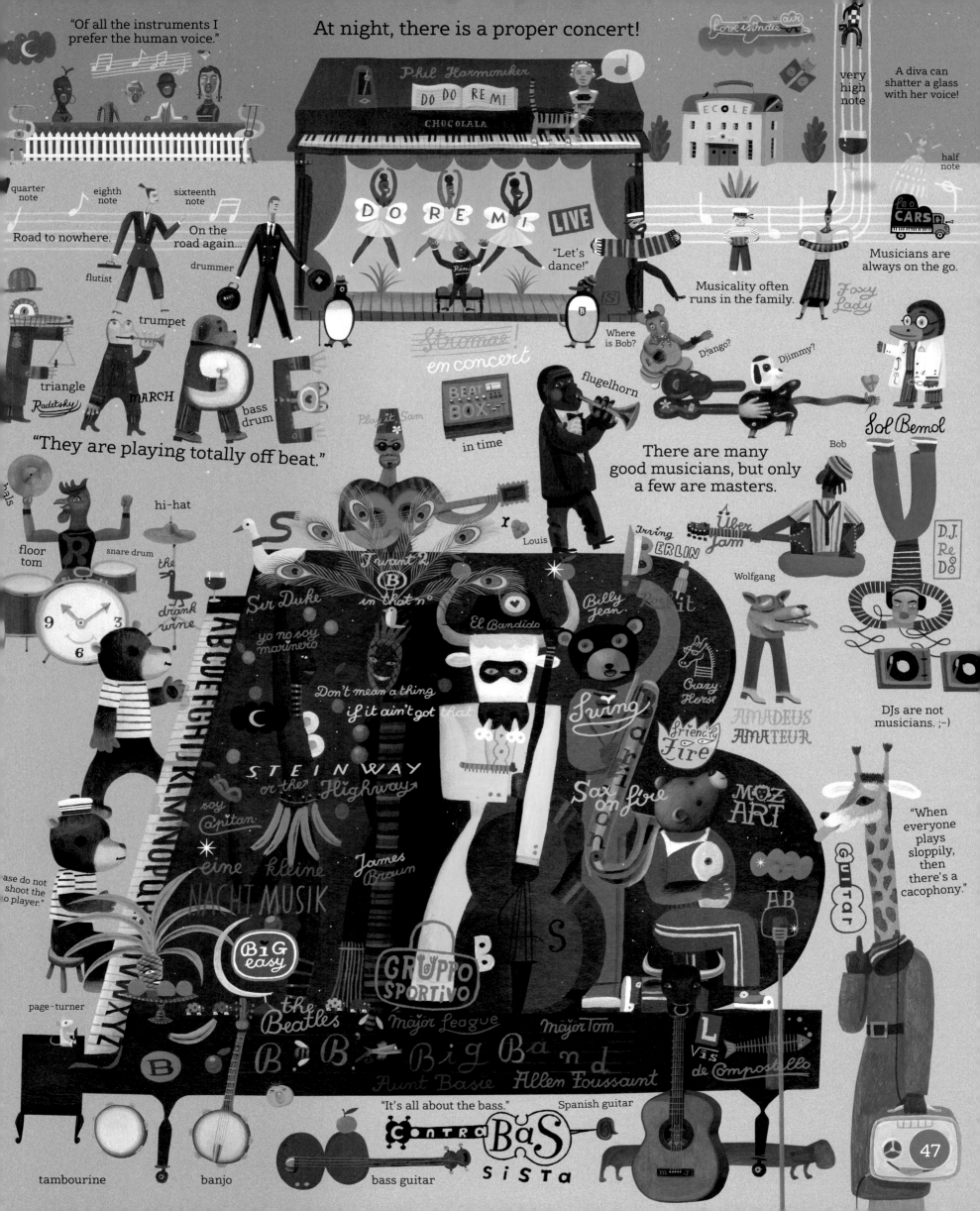

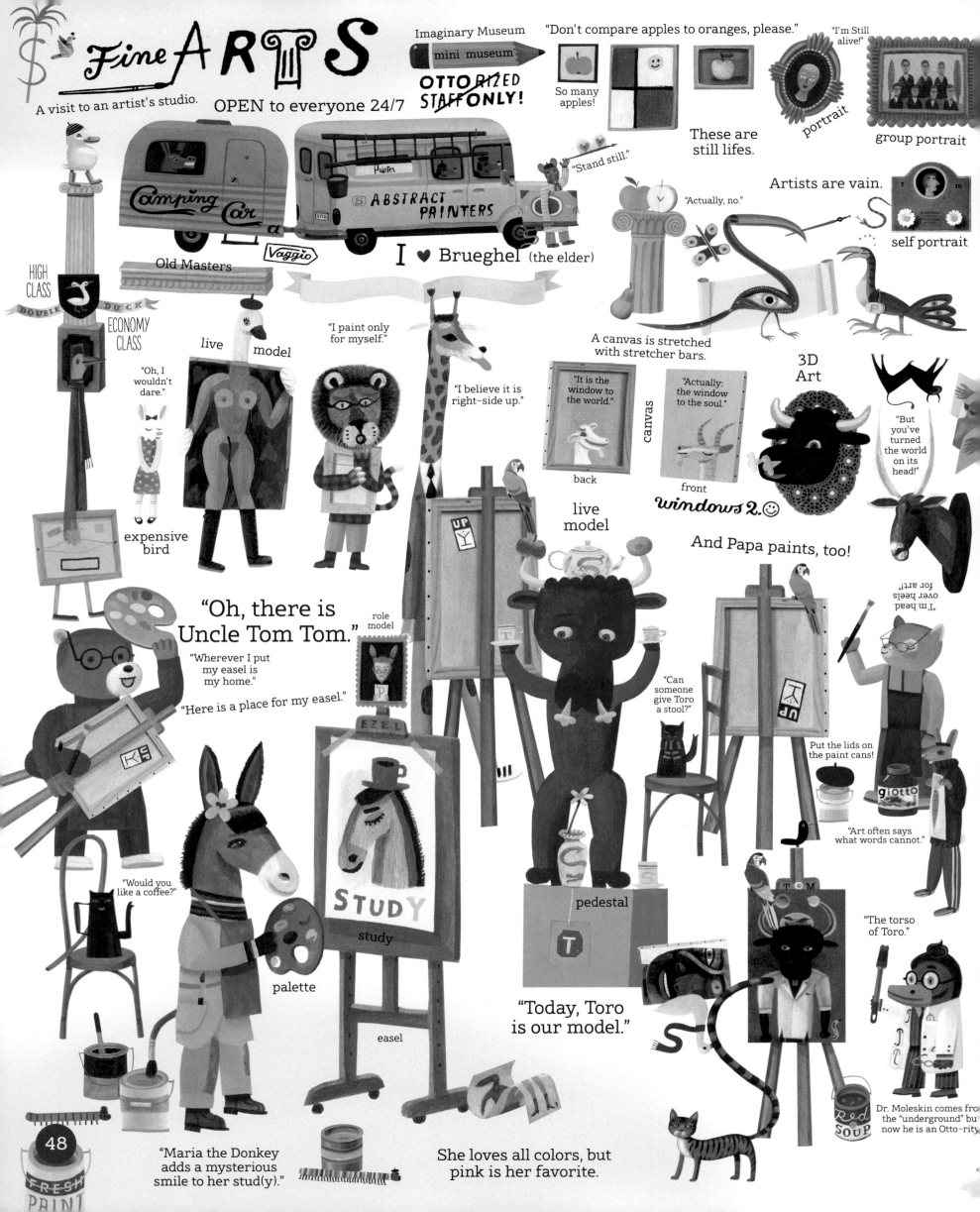

Fine ARTS

A visit to an artist's studio.
OPEN to everyone 24/7

Imaginary Museum
mini museum
OTTORIZED STAFF ONLY!

"Don't compare apples to oranges, please."

So many apples!

These are still lifes.

"I'm Still alive!"

portrait

group portrait

Old Masters

Camping Car
Vaggio

"Stand still."

ABSTRACT PAINTERS
Painter

I ♥ Brueghel (the elder)

Artists are vain.

"Actually, no."

self portrait

HIGH CLASS

DOUBLE DUCK

ECONOMY CLASS

"Oh, I wouldn't dare."

live model

"I paint only for myself."

"I believe it is right-side up."

A canvas is stretched with stretcher bars.

3D Art

"It is the window to the world."

"Actually: the window to the soul."

canvas

back

front

windows 2. ☺

"But you've turned the world on its head!"

expensive bird

"Oh, there is Uncle Tom Tom."

role model

"Wherever I put my easel is my home."

"Here is a place for my easel."

live model

And Papa paints, too!

"I'm head over heels for art!"

"Can someone give Toro a stool?"

Put the lids on the paint cans!

giotto

"Art often says what words cannot."

EZEL

STUDY

"Would you like a coffee?"

palette

study

easel

pedestal

"Today, Toro is our model."

"The torso of Toro."

Red SOUP

Dr. Moleskin comes from the "underground" but now he is an Otto-rity.

48

"Maria the Donkey adds a mysterious smile to her stud(y)."

FRESH PAINT

She loves all colors, but pink is her favorite.

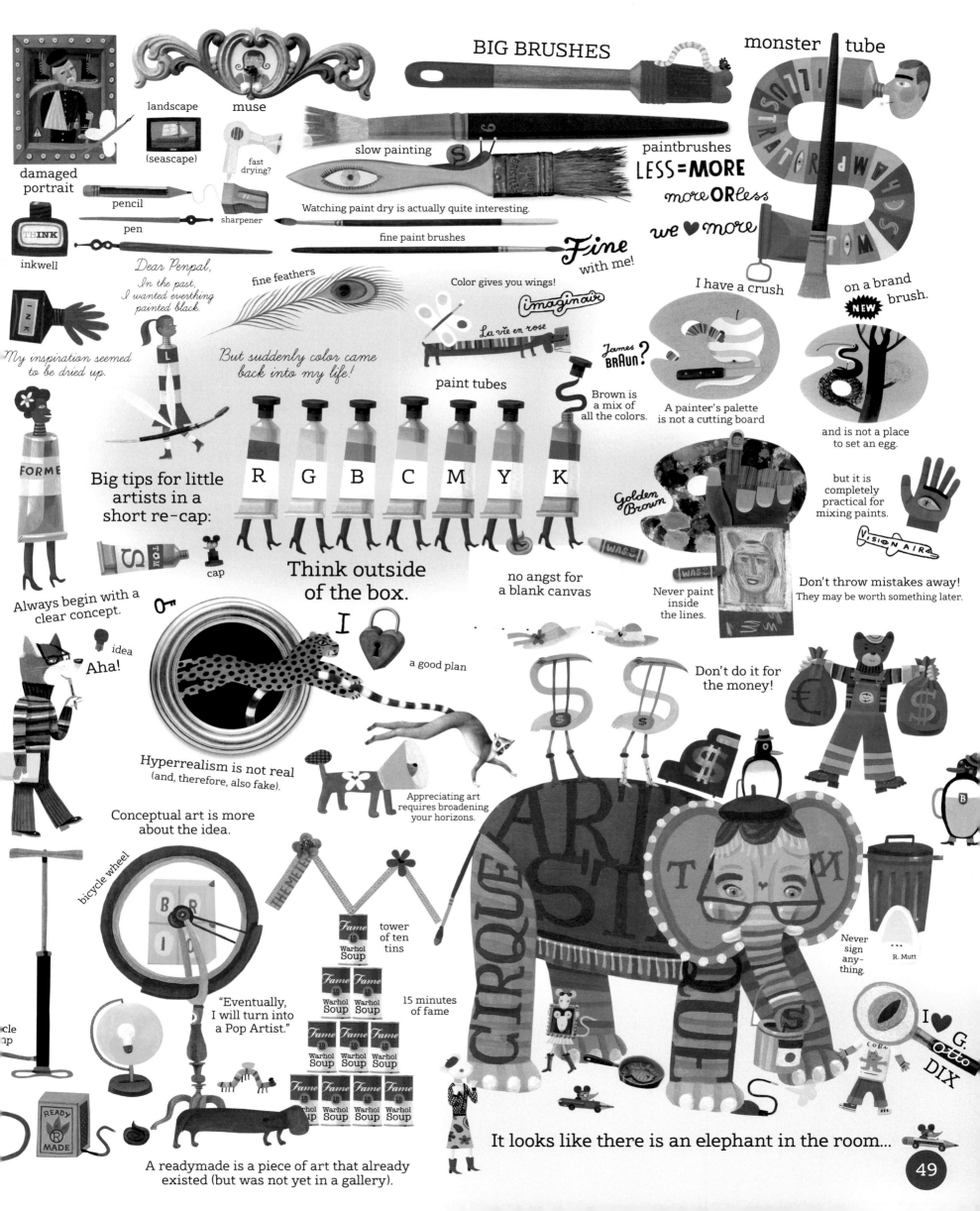

BIG BRUSHES

monster tube

landscape

muse

damaged portrait

(seascape)

fast drying?

slow painting

pencil

pen

sharpener

inkwell

Watching paint dry is actually quite interesting.

fine paint brushes

paintbrushes

LESS = MORE

more OR less

we ♥ more

Fine with me!

THINK

I have a crush

on a brand NEW brush.

Dear Penpal,
In the past,
I wanted everything
painted black.

fine feathers

Color gives you wings!

imaginair

La vie en rose

My inspiration seemed
to be dried up.

But suddenly color came
back into my life!

paint tubes

James BRAUN?

Brown is
a mix of
all the colors.

A painter's palette
is not a cutting board

and is not a place
to set an egg.

FORME

Big tips for little
artists in a
short re-cap:

R G B C M Y K

Golden Brown

but it is
completely
practical for
mixing paints.

VISIONAIR

cap

Think outside
of the box.

no angst for
a blank canvas

Never paint
inside
the lines.

Don't throw mistakes away!
They may be worth something later.

Always begin with a
clear concept.

idea
Aha!

a good plan

Don't do it for
the money!

Hyperrealism is not real
(and, therefore, also fake).

Conceptual art is more
about the idea.

Appreciating art
requires broadening
your horizons.

bicycle wheel

Fame
Warhol
Soup

tower
of ten
tins

15 minutes
of fame

CIRQUE ARTIST

Never
sign
any-
thing.

R. Mutt

I ♥ G. Otto DIX

"Eventually,
I will turn into
a Pop Artist."

Fame
Warhol Soup

Fame
Warhol Soup

Fame
Warhol
Soup

Fame
Warhol
Soup

Fame
Warhol
Soup

Fame
Warhol
Soup

Fame
Warhol
Soup

Fame
Warhol
Soup

READY
R MADE

A readymade is a piece of art that already
existed (but was not yet in a gallery).

It looks like there is an elephant in the room...

49

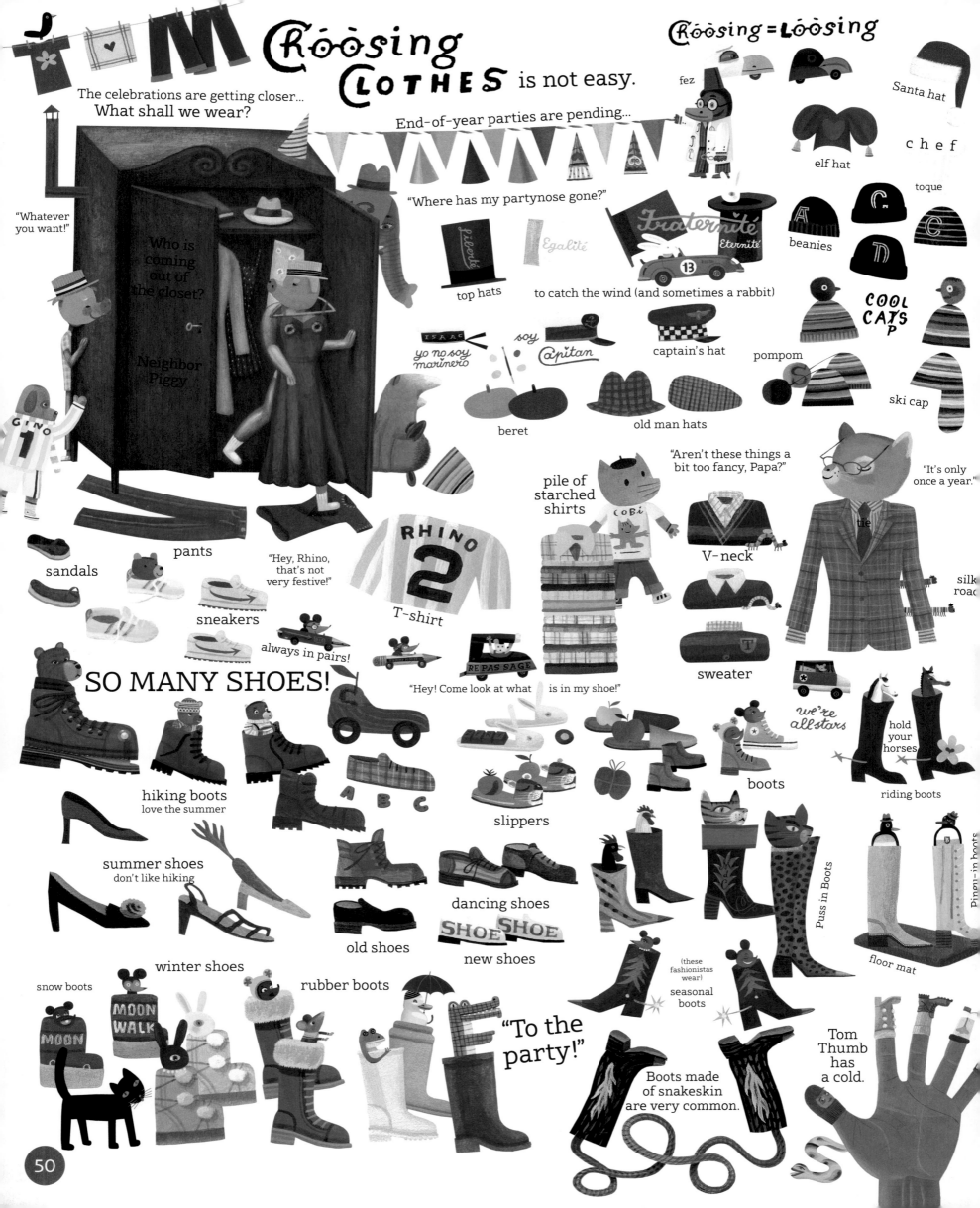

TOM

CHOOSING CLOTHES is not easy.

CHOOSING = LOOSING

The celebrations are getting closer...
What shall we wear?

End-of-year parties are pending...

"Where has my partynose gone?"

"Whatever you want!"

Who is coming out of the closet?

Neighbor Piggy

GINO 1

fez

Santa hat

elf hat

c h e f

toque

beanies

A G C D

COOL CATS P

top hats

Liberté   Egalité   Fraternité Eternité

to catch the wind (and sometimes a rabbit)

13

ISAAC
yo no soy marinero   soy Capitan

captain's hat

pompom

ski cap

beret   old man hats

"Aren't these things a bit too fancy, Papa?"

"It's only once a year."

pile of starched shirts

COBI

V-neck

tie

silk road

sandals   pants

"Hey, Rhino, that's not very festive!"

RHINO 2

T-shirt

sneakers

always in pairs!

SO MANY SHOES!

RE PAS SAGE

"Hey! Come look at what is in my shoe!"

sweater

we're all stars

hold your horses

hiking boots
love the summer

A B C

slippers

boots

riding boots

summer shoes
don't like hiking

dancing shoes

SHOE SHOE

old shoes

new shoes

Puss in Boots

floor mat

winter shoes

snow boots

MOON   MOON WALK

rubber boots

"To the party!"

(these fashionistas wear)
seasonal boots

Boots made of snakeskin are very common.

Tom Thumb has a cold.

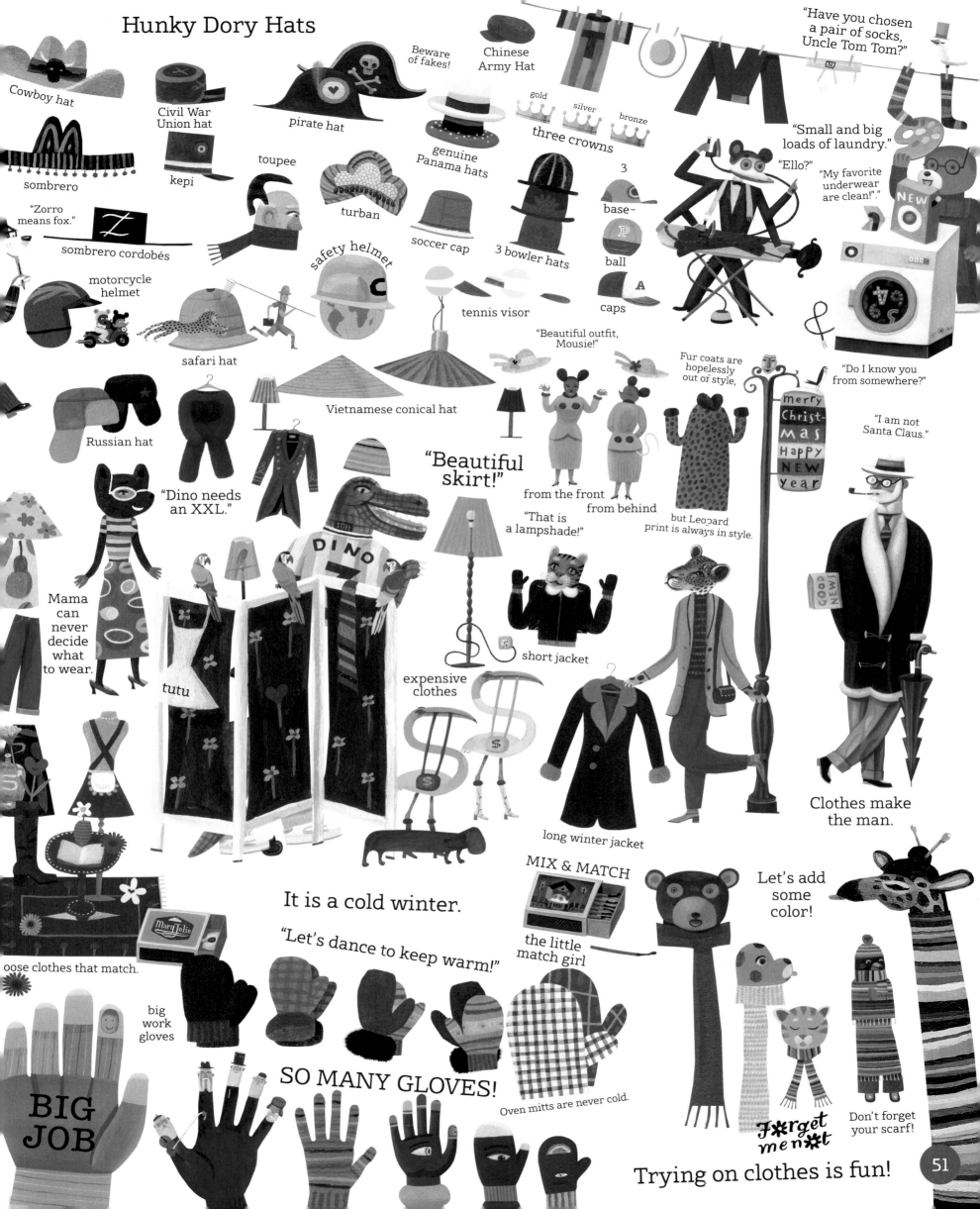

Hunky Dory Hats

Cowboy hat

Civil War Union hat

Beware of fakes!

pirate hat

Chinese Army Hat

sombrero

kepi

toupee

genuine Panama hats

gold   silver   bronze

three crowns

turban

3 base-ball caps

"Zorro means fox."

sombrero cordobés

safety helmet

soccer cap

3 bowler hats

tennis visor

motorcycle helmet

safari hat

Vietnamese conical hat

"Have you chosen a pair of socks, Uncle Tom Tom?"

"Small and big loads of laundry."

"Ello?"

"My favorite underwear are clean!"."

"Do I know you from somewhere?"

"I am not Santa Claus."

"Beautiful outfit, Mousie!"

Fur coats are hopelessly out of style,

merry Christ-mas Happy NEW year

from the front

from behind

but Leopard print is always in style.

Russian hat

"Dino needs an XXL."

"Beautiful skirt!"

"That is a lampshade!"

DINO

short jacket

Mama can never decide what to wear.

tutu

expensive clothes

GOOD NEWS

Clothes make the man.

long winter jacket

It is a cold winter.

oose clothes that match.

"Let's dance to keep warm!"

MIX & MATCH

the little match girl

Let's add some color!

MaryJolie

BIG JOB

big work gloves

SO MANY GLOVES!

Oven mitts are never cold.

Forget me not

Don't forget your scarf!

Trying on clothes is fun!

51

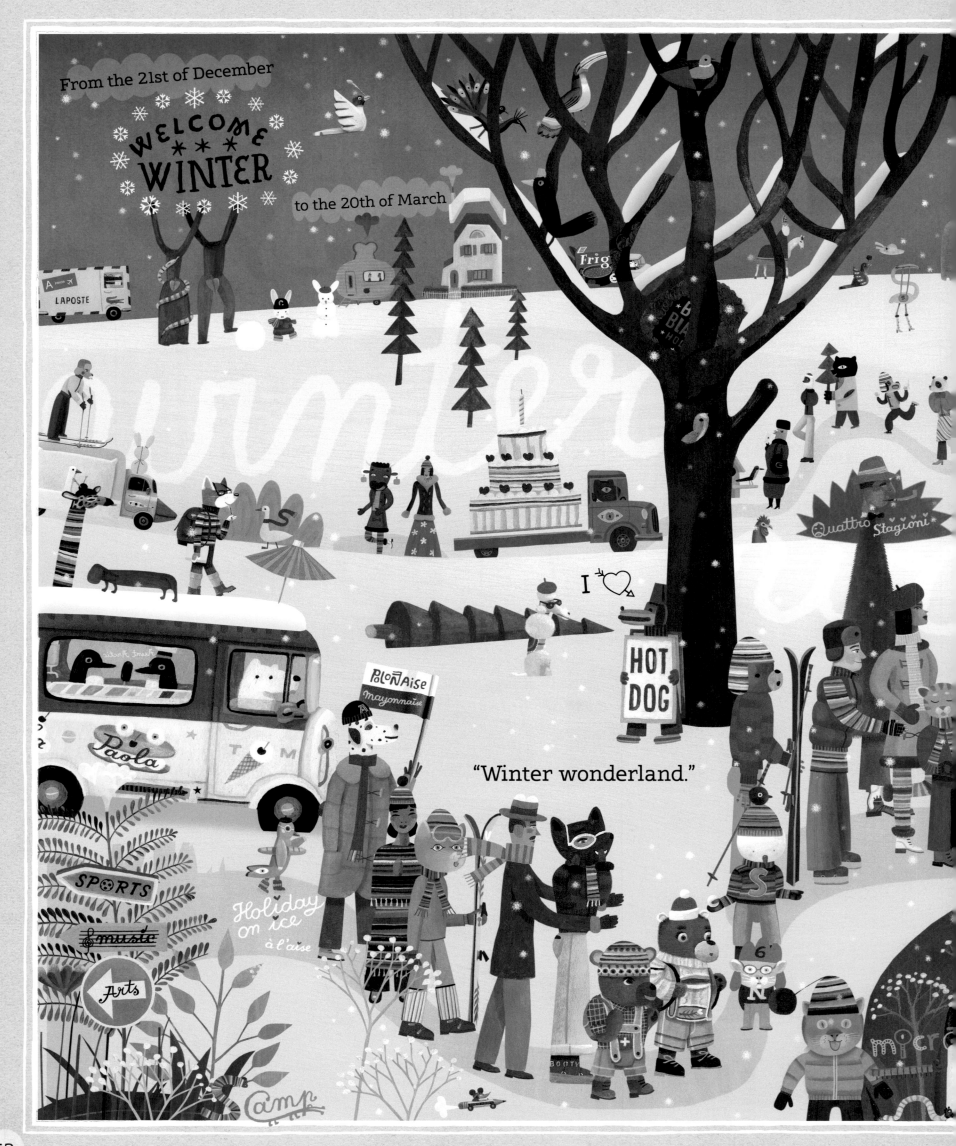

From the 21st of December
to the 20th of March

WELCOME WINTER

"Winter wonderland."

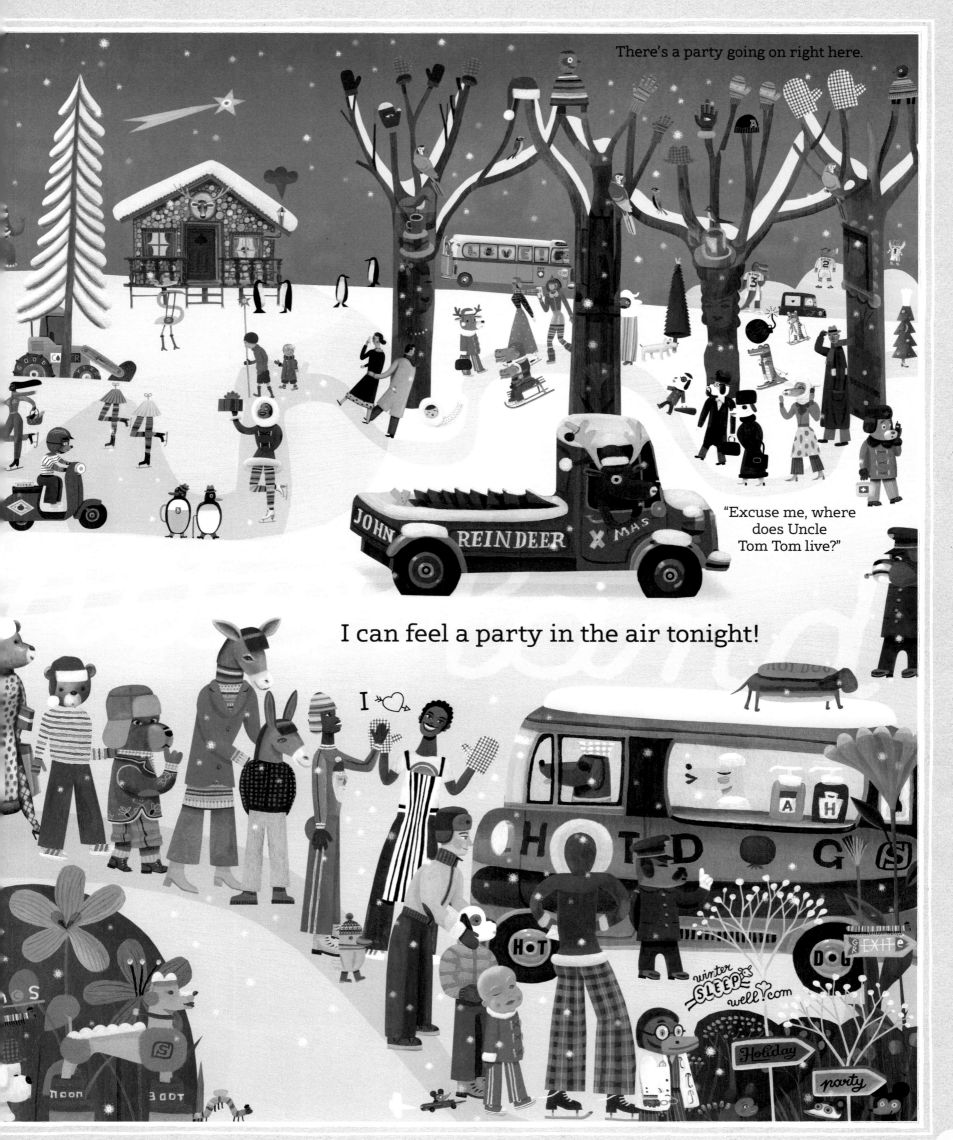

There's a party going on right here.

"Excuse me, where does Uncle Tom Tom live?"

I can feel a party in the air tonight!

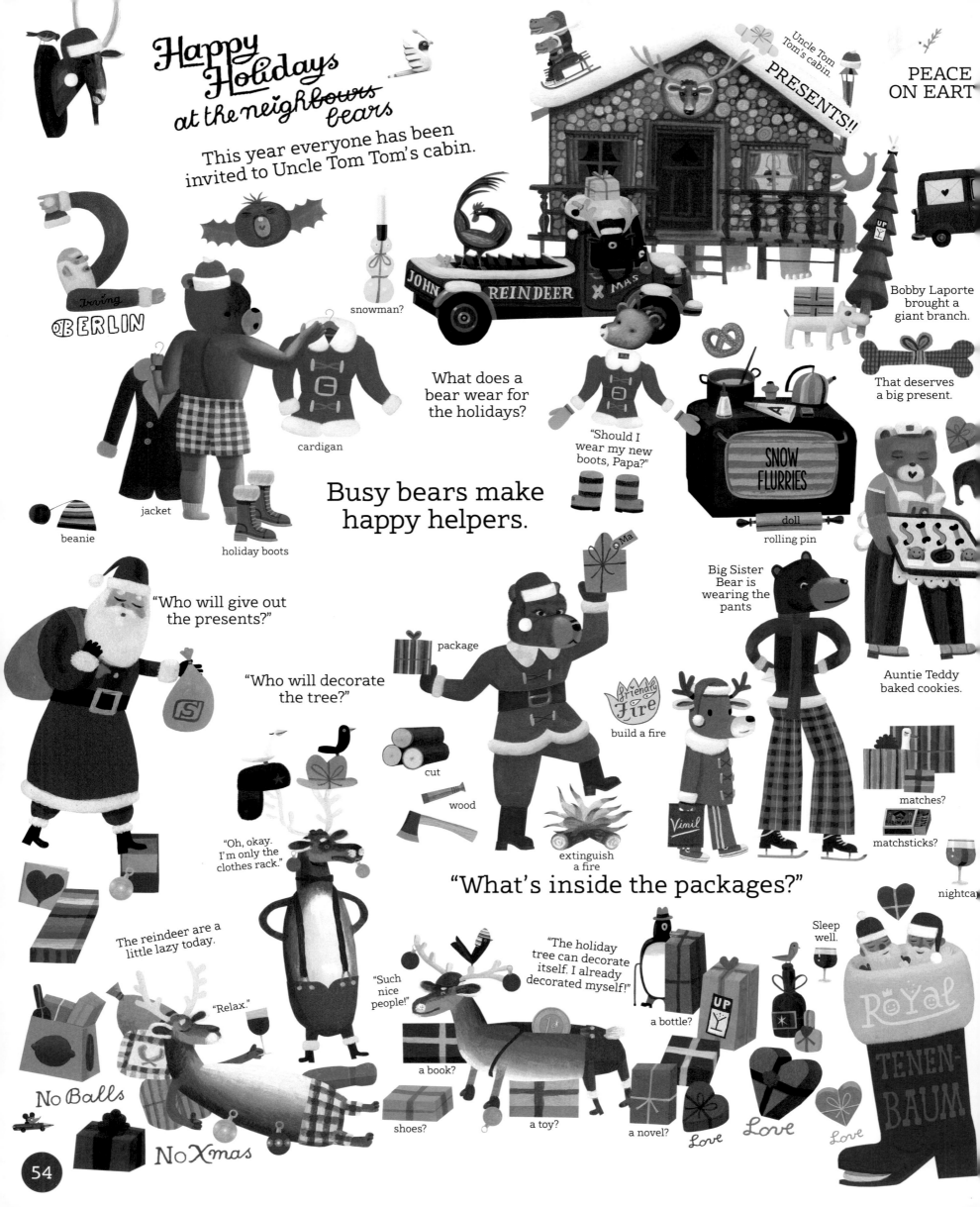

Happy Holidays at the neighbours bears

This year everyone has been invited to Uncle Tom Tom's cabin.

PEACE ON EART

Uncle Tom Tom's cabin.

PRESENTS!!

BERLIN
Irving

snowman?

JOHN REINDEER XMAS

What does a bear wear for the holidays?

"Should I wear my new boots, Papa?"

SNOW FLURRIES

Bobby Laporte brought a giant branch.

That deserves a big present.

cardigan

jacket

beanie

holiday boots

Busy bears make happy helpers.

doll

rolling pin

Big Sister Bear is wearing the pants

Auntie Teddy baked cookies.

"Who will give out the presents?"

"Who will decorate the tree?"

package

O Ma

Friendly Fire

build a fire

matches?

matchsticks?

nightca

"Oh, okay. I'm only the clothes rack."

cut

wood

extinguish a fire

Vimil

"What's inside the packages?"

The reindeer are a little lazy today.

"Relax."

"Such nice people!"

"The holiday tree can decorate itself. I already decorated myself!"

Sleep well.

a bottle?

a book?

No Balls

No Xmas

shoes?

a toy?

a novel?

Love

Love

Love

ROYAL

TENEN-BAUM

54

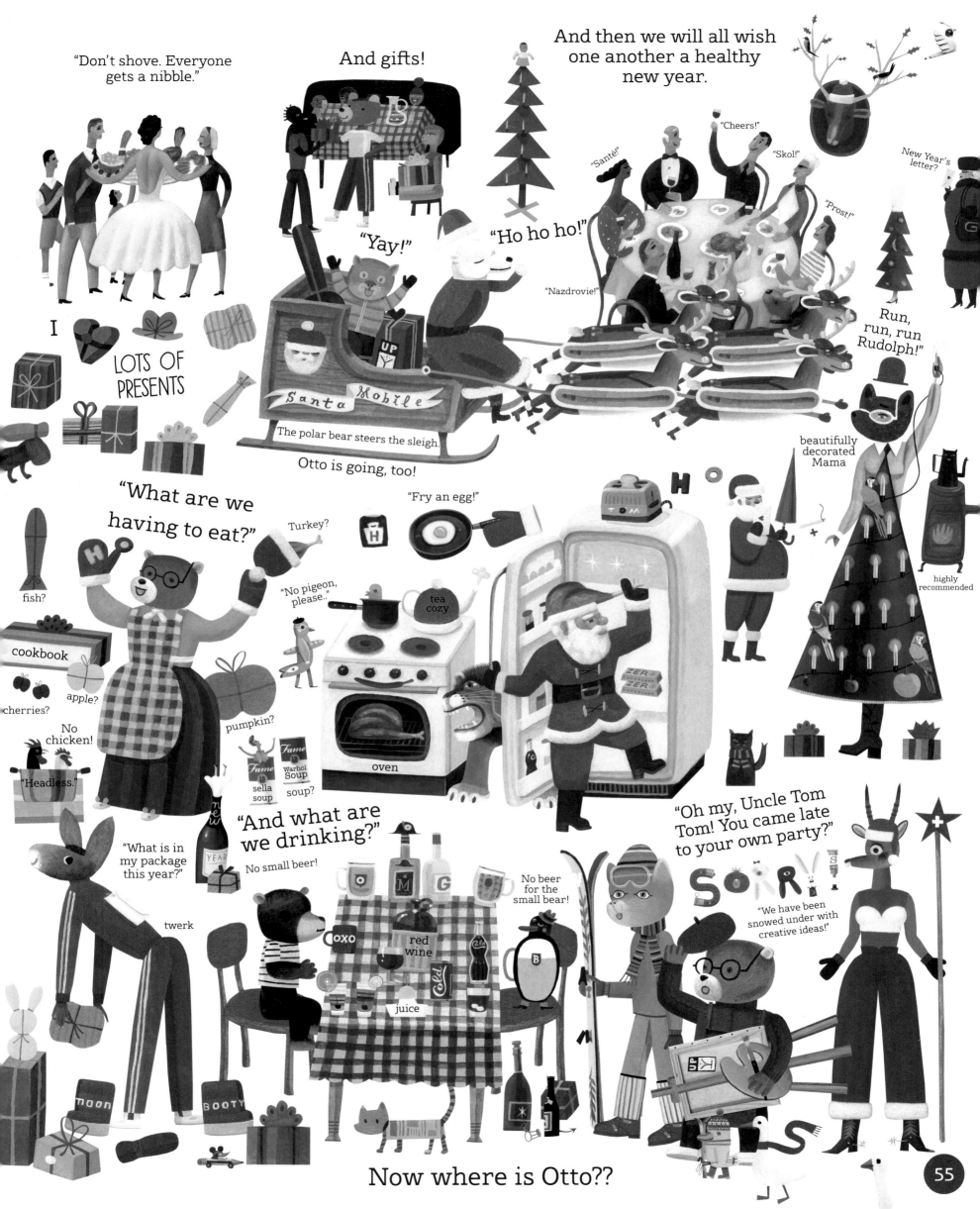

New Year! The concert hall is completely finished! The book is almost finished...

The world is small.

The world is big.

And the universe is even bigger.

"Time for bed, Otto."

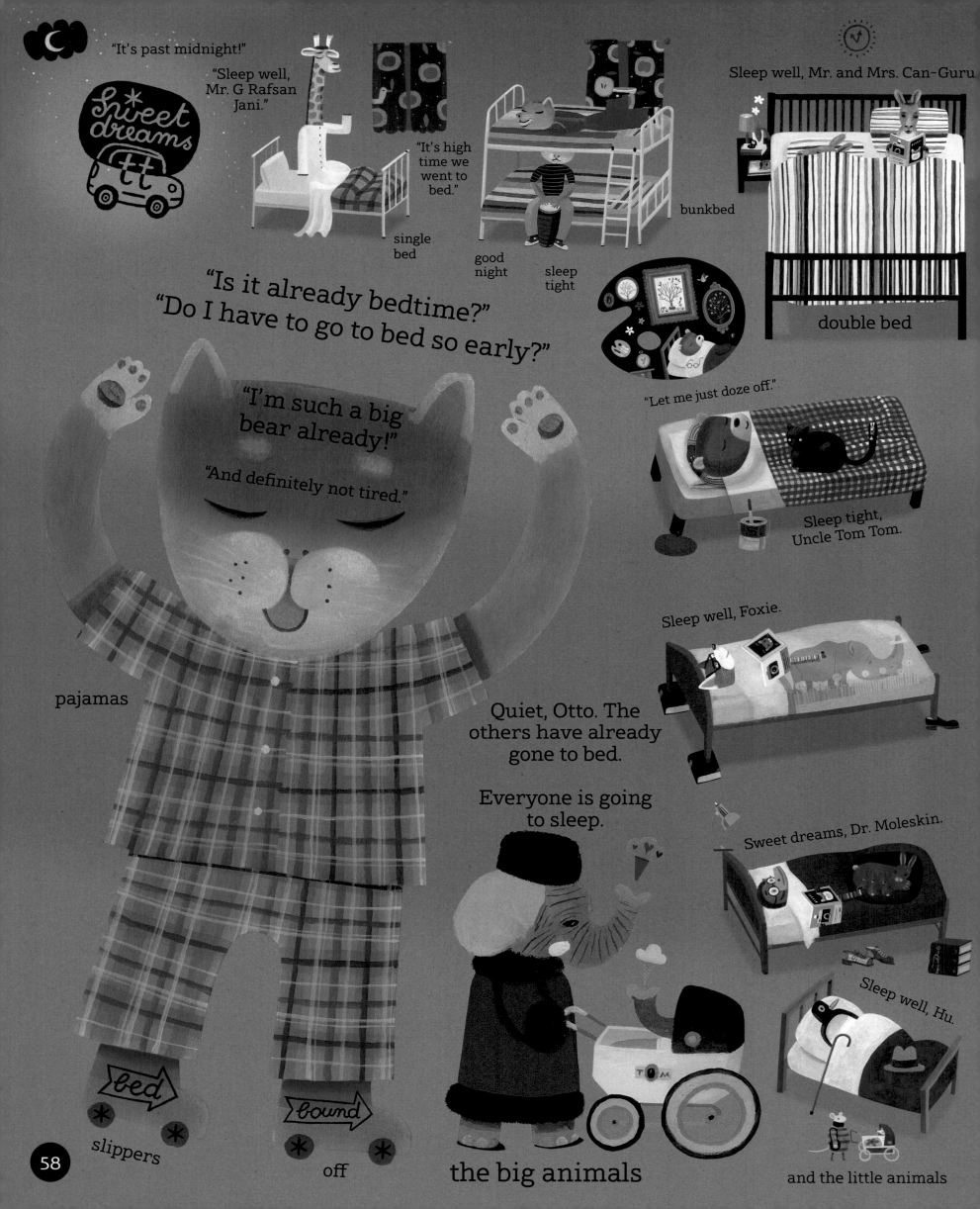

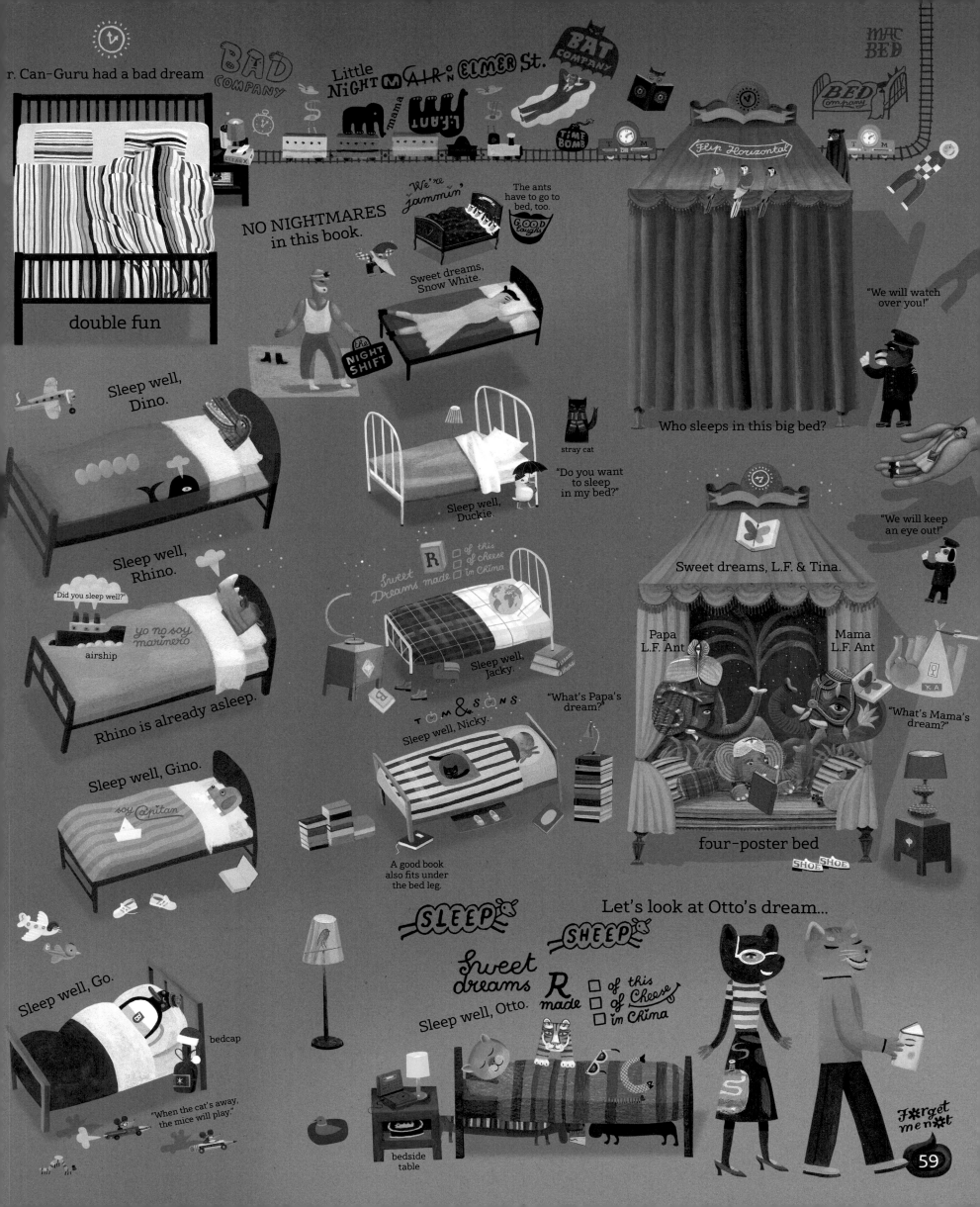

r. Can-Guru had a bad dream

BAD COMPANY

Little Night MARE ON ELMER St.

Mama L.F. ant

BAT COMPANY

TIME BOMB

MAC BED

BED Company

double fun

NO NIGHTMARES in this book.

We're jammin'

The ants have to go to bed, too.

GOOD laughs

Sweet dreams, Snow White.

the NIGHT SHIFT

Flip Horizontal

"We will watch over you!"

Sleep well, Dino.

Who sleeps in this big bed?

stray cat

"Do you want to sleep in my bed?"

Sleep well, Duckie.

"We will keep an eye out!"

Sleep well, Rhino.

"Did you sleep well?"

yo no soy marinero

airship

Sweet Dreams made R □ of this □ of Cheese □ in China

Sleep well, Jacky.

Sweet dreams, L.F. & Tina.

Papa L.F. Ant

Mama L.F. Ant

Rhino is already asleep.

TOM & SONS

"What's Papa's dream?"

"What's Mama's dream?"

Sleep well, Gino.

soy Capitan

Sleep well, Nicky.

A good book also fits under the bed leg.

four-poster bed

SHOE SHOE

SLEEP SHEEP

Let's look at Otto's dream...

Sweet dreams

R made □ of this □ of Cheese □ in China

Sleep well, Go.

Sleep well, Otto.

bedcap

"When the cat's away, the mice will play."

bedside table

Forget me not

59

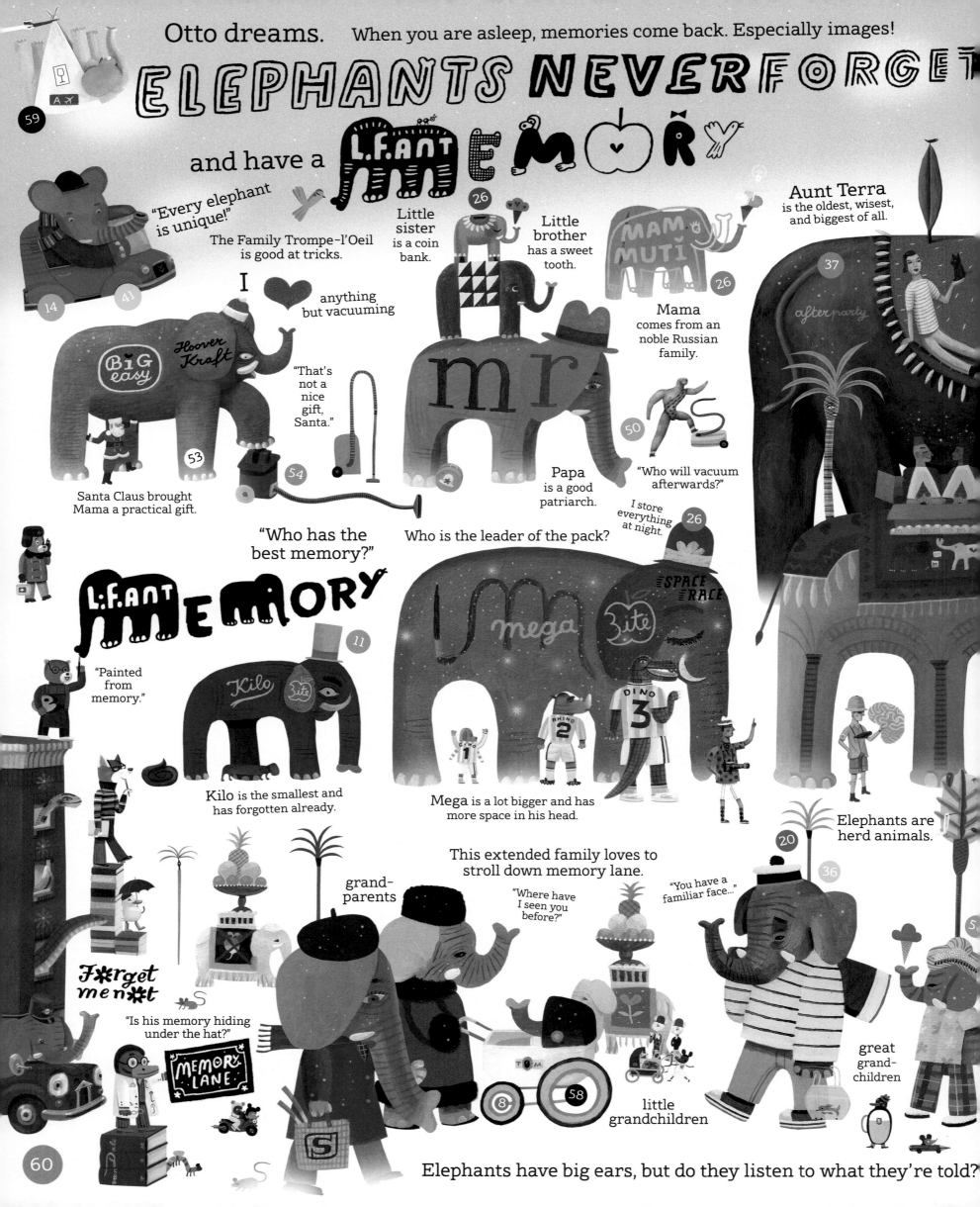

Otto dreams. When you are asleep, memories come back. Especially images!

ELEPHANTS NEVER FORGET

and have a L.F.ANT MEMORY

"Every elephant is unique!"

The Family Trompe-l'Oeil is good at tricks.

Little sister is a coin bank.

Little brother has a sweet tooth.

MAM MUTI

Aunt Terra is the oldest, wisest, and biggest of all.

I ♥ anything but vacuuming

BiG easy Hoover Kraft

"That's not a nice gift, Santa."

mr

Mama comes from an noble Russian family.

Santa Claus brought Mama a practical gift.

Papa is a good patriarch.

"Who will vacuum afterwards?"

I store everything at night.

"Who has the best memory?"

Who is the leader of the pack?

L.F.ANT MEMORY

"Painted from memory."

Kilo 3ite

mega 3ite

SPACE RACE

Kilo is the smallest and has forgotten already.

RHINO 2

DINO 3

Mega is a lot bigger and has more space in his head.

Elephants are herd animals.

Forget me not

This extended family loves to stroll down memory lane.

grand-parents

"Where have I seen you before?"

"You have a familiar face..."

"Is his memory hiding under the hat?"

MEMORY LANE

TOM

little grandchildren

great grand-children

Elephants have big ears, but do they listen to what they're told?

Giga Bite

L.F.ANTS ... N PARADE

DESSERT

does what he wants (is actually smaller than Terra).

Terra is very fond of children.

Giga has a gigantic ego. ;)

Couch Potato

SEAT SNIFFER

TOM

Elephants are BIG

Cats and mice are rather small.

eine kleine NACHT PIANOELEPHANT MUSIK

Igor and Ivor are always up for a bit of music.

made of Cheese

Sweet dreams

hope for the best prepare for the worst

CIRQUE ARTISTE

In the past, Tomasito was fooled by two birds who promised him fame and fortune.

Circus elephants used to come from India.

And one more little elephant with a long trunk and...

MIND YOUR HAT

Fin

"It looks like an elephant graveyard!"

... our picture book is finished!

en Fin

Red SOUP

How many elephants are there on these two pages?

You need an elephant's patience.

61

Do you know these countries??

Canada

USA

Formula 1

Great Britain

The Netherlands

BYE, MICE

Trinidad

Puerto Rico

Cuba

Hasta Siempre

Guantanamera

Tobago

Jamaica

SUPER

Belgium

We *Jammin'*

Double Czech

Czech Republic

AIR JORDANS

Palestine

Hungary

Szia!

MAGYAR POSTA

ILLUZIONIST

We're *Jahmen!*

Germany

WIRTSCHAFT WUNDER

Wir schaffen das

BERLIN

Mexico

Portugal

Vinho Verde

ABRAÇO!

Spain

olé

Italy

Ciao Bella

Arrivederci.

Israel

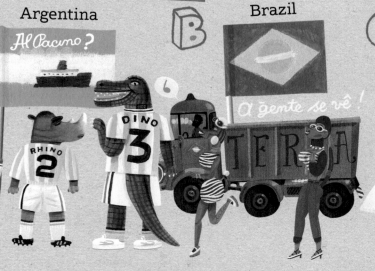 Argentina

Al Pacino?

Don't cry 4 me

RHINO 2

DINO 3

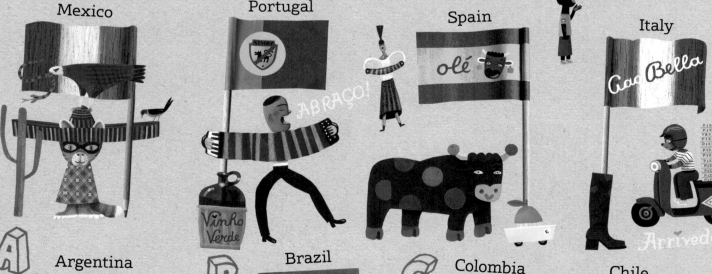 Brazil

A gente se vê!

TERRA

Colombia

Christophorus

Colombus

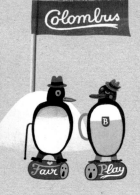 Chile

Con Carne?

TOM

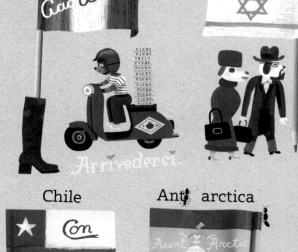 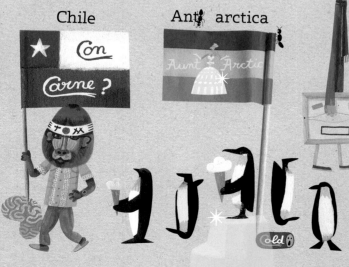 Ant arctica

Aunt Arctica

old